MEDICAL INJURY CLAIMS

IN THE NETHERLANDS

Medical Injury Claims in The Netherlands

A survey of the settlement of medical injury claims by Dutch insurers during the period 1980–1990

Joseph H. Hubben
Leontine G. Angenent

Faculty of Law
University of Nijmegen

CRC Press
Taylor & Francis Group
Boca Raton London New York

CRC Press is an imprint of the
Taylor & Francis Group, an **informa** business
A TAYLOR & FRANCIS BOOK

Medical Injury Claims in The Netherlands is an English translation of Medische schadeclaims in Nederland 1980-1990 University of Nijmegen, Faculty of Law Recht en Samenleving nr 6 Nijmegen 1992

First published 1996 by Taylor & Francis.

Published 2023 by CRC Press
Taylor & Francis Group
6000 Broken Sound Parkway NW, Suite 300
Boca Raton, FL 33487-2742

ISBN-13: 978-90-70430-17-7 (hbk)

Publisher's Note
The publisher has gone to lengths to ensure the quality of this reprint but points out that some imperfections in the original copies may be apparent.

Visit the Taylor & Francis Web site at
http://www.taylorandfrancis.com

and the CRC Press Web site at
http://www.crcpress.com

CONTENTS

FOREWORD

Relatively little has been known up to now about the settlement of medical injury claims by Dutch insurers, and it is hoped that this survey and the report based on it will fill this gap. Because of the co-operation of the insurance companies who belonged to the former M.A.R. group and Centraal Beheer, it has been possible to conduct a wide-ranging case survey of the way in which medical injury claims in hospitals are settled.

This extensive survey was supported by the Dutch Ministry of National Health, Welfare and Sports.
A valuable contribution to the survey was also made by M. Heineman and M. van Cruchten. Furthermore, we gratefully acknowledge the benefit we received from the advice given by A. Kroonen, a medical practitioner affiliated with the Institute for Social Medicine, University of Nijmegen, and J. van der Putten, Department of Methods and Techniques, Faculty of Social Sciences, University of Nijmegen.

This survey was published in Dutch in 1992

Nijmegen, September 1995

J.H. Hubben
L.G. Angenent

Chapter 1

Introduction and Reasons for the Survey

The subject of medical liability in the Netherlands is very much in a state of flux, a situation which may be illustrated by the Medical Treatment Agreements bill, which, among other things, introduced a central liability for hospitals. Moreover, on 1st January 1992 Volume 6 of the New Civil Code came into force. This section of the Code contains a number of new rules concerning, *inter alia*, unforeseen circumstances and a check on the level of indemnities. And quite apart from this, there are other developments connected with European legislation, which has already obliged us to introduce a new regulation in respect of product liability. Of additional importance in this connection is the discussion about the so called patients' injuries insurance and the legal measure, announced by the government, concerning the right of public health service-related complaints. We must also refer in this context to the widening of the definition of the term "loss"[1].

In assessing the consequences of these developments, it is extremely important to realise the way in which injury claims for medical injuries in the Netherlands are settled. Up to the present time there has been hardly any understanding of this subject. The department of Health Law at the University of Nijmegen had earlier conducted a limited survey of cases dealt with by the *Centraal Beheer* insurance company. This investigation covered 197 injury claims which had been made during the years 1980 to 1988 inclusive and which had been concluded by the end of 1988. The results were published in 1989[2]. The limited extent of this survey, however, permitted no general conclusions to be drawn.

In 1990 the survey was extended to the reinsurance group *Medische Aansprakelijkheidsrisico's (M.A.R.)*[3]. At the same time the *Centraal Beheer* survey was continued on a larger scale. Both companies gave their full co-

---

[1] The Dutch "schade" (=*damnum*) is translated variously, according to context, as "loss", "injury", "damage", "claim".

[2] J.H. Hubben and L.G. Angenent, Settlement of Medical Injury claims. In: Rechtsbijstand in de gezondheidszorg (ed. J.H. Hubben), 1989, pp. 9-23.

[3] Meaning "Medical Liability Risks".

operation in the conduct of this extensive survey, which provides a picture of the settlement of medical injury claims in the Netherlands.

The survey involved those insurance companies which had been members of the *Medische Aansprakelijkheidsrisico's* reinsurance group *(M.A.R.)*, which had existed down to the middle of 1991, and the *Centraal Beheer* insurance company. The *M.A.R.* was a large reinsurer of medical liability risks. This reinsurance pool was set up in 1977. On the basis of a mutual reinsurance the sixteen affiliated companies undertook to pay a premium related to the market share of each individual company. At the time the group included the following companies: *Nationale Nederlanden, Winterthur, Centraal Beheer, VVAA, UAP, Tollenaar & Wegener, AEGON, De Centrale, Delta Lloyd and Royal Nederland.*

In addition to trying to achieve a better spread of the risk, the aims of the *M.A.R.* included an attempt to achieve uniformity of liability and claims settlement, on the one hand, and of a policy regarding conditions and acceptance, on the other, as well as the promotion of claim prevention. During the eighties a number of companies withdrew from the *M.A.R.*, usually citing as the most important reason for their departure the fact that the risk was too great or the market segment too small.

As mentioned, the *M.A.R.* continued in existence as a reinsurer until July 1991. Since that time the companies formerly affiliated to it have again been conducting an independent policy concerning medical liability risks. In 1980 *Centraal Beheer* started offering insurance policies in the care sector on an independent basis.

These companies together insure some 80% of Dutch hospitals. The survey covers the period from 1980 to 1990, the last day of 1990 being taken as the reference date. During this ten-year period a total of 3970 injury claims were submitted for medical injuries sustained in hospitals.

An injury claim was included in the survey if it met the following conditions:

1. the injury occurred in a general or university hospital (not a nursinghome, psychiatric hospital, general practice etc.);

2. the injury was suffered by the patient and a third party possibly also suffers an indirect loss (sickness costs insurance, employer etc.); the survey does not cover injuries suffered by hospital staff or visitors;

3. the loss consists of damage caused by the injury (not a mere financial or property loss; lost spectacles, dentures etc. fall outside the scope of the

survey, as do also pure financial losses suffered by a business based on damage to reputation);

4. the injury is related to the treatment. This criterion embraces not just treatment by a doctor, but may also include acts committed by a nurse, analyst, physiotherapist etc.; for example, injury-related damage due to an accident involving a lift or a revolving door is not covered;

5. the injury is reported during the period 1980 to 1989, both years included.

During the period covered by the survey 495 medical injury claims meeting the above criteria were made to *Centraal Beheer* and are all included in the survey. The number of medical injury claims made to the *M.A.R.* during this period comes to approx. 3475. Using a random non-selective procedure, we chose 1158 cases (1 in 3) for inclusion in the survey. It emerged that these 1158 cases, taken together, contained 1224 claims; 1 case refers to 54 claims by women who contracted hepatitis B following *in vitro* fertilisation treatment with an infected serum; one case contains 12 claims relating to injuries suffered as a result of radiation from the use of unsound equipment. In addition, there is one case which covers two claims relating to incorrect obstetric assistance being administered on two occasions during confinement.
Finally, there is one case containing two claims by haemophiliac patients who became infected with the HIV virus through the administration of blood products.

From the 1224 cases selected, 110 claims have been excluded from the survey because they do not involve injuries but refer to property damage. Moreover, 59 of the cases selected for the samples taken at random cannot now be traced. These cases appear principally to have been reported during the years 1981-1986. Hence, there are 1055 medical liability cases still available for the survey. The statement by the *M.A.R.* explaining the fact that 59 cases can no longer be traced means that the majority of them involve cases which, although they may indeed be regarded as referring to injury-related damage, have had a time limit put on them as though they were property claims (three years). According to the *M.A.R.*, these involve minor injury claims, viz. dental lesions. Moreover, since 1st January 1992 the major companies who had earlier been affiliated to the *M.A.R.* have (once again) been treating damage to dentures as property damage.

To summarise, 1550 injury claims were investigated, of which 1055 cases originated from the *M.A.R.* (drawn from a non-selective random sample) and 495 (the whole population) from *Centraal Beheer*. Hence, we have a data matrix of n = 1550 injury claims.
In granting their consent to the survey, the insurers stipulated certain

restrictions. As a result, the survey omitted any qualitative assessment of the manner in which the claims in question were settled. Moreover, no inspection was allowed of the medical files which were drawn up alongside the claims files.

The survey was carried out with the aid of a questionnaire drawn up in consultation with the insurers. In the main, this contains questions of a financial nature (e.g. size of the claim, level of indemnity paid, compensation for pain and suffering), and legal aspects (the position with regard to liability, legal assistance, civil and disciplinary law procedures etc.), the social characteristics of those who had made injury claims and the medical aspects (including classification of the operation, the type of operator, injury and medical context). A doctor was consulted for the assessment of the medical aspects appearing in the claims file.

Because the *Centraal Beheer* data refer to the whole population, while those from the *M.A.R.* represent only a random sample, when the survey material had been collected we looked to see whether, on any crucial points, the *M.A.R.* data remained within the 90% confidence intervals. This transpired always to be the case. On the strength of this finding it was decided to merge the data from both insurers into one data matrix, which means that the percentages given in the report are common to both *M.A.R.* and *Centraal Beheer.*
Where absolute figures are given they refer to the data in the data matrix (n = 1550). If one wishes to calculate absolute figures for the *M.A.R.* and *Centraal Beheer* populations separately, then the *M.A.R.* and *Centraal Beheer* material will have to be split. Next a confidence interval around the numbers found in the random sample will have to be introduced for the *M.A.R.* data, on the basis of which, finally, a population estimate can be made.

Of the 1550 cases included in the survey, 1296 had been concluded by the reference date (31-12-1990), while 252 are still pending. In two cases the status of a file was uncertain.

The survey concerned itself firstly with the question of how injury claims made by patients[4] as a result of incidents in hospitals are settled. In how many cases is an indemnity paid and is there a certain trend to be observed in the level of indemnities paid to patients? Is it true that the number of injury claims is rising and is this also true for the number of cases in which the patient receives an indemnity?

---

4 For the sake of simplicity it is assumed in the text that it is the patient who has made the claim. Table 23, however, shows that other persons do this as well.

Chapter 2

THE FINANCIAL ASPECTS

How has the number of injury claims made to insurers during the period covered by the survey grown? This trend is shown in the graph below (figure 1), which provides an overview of the number of injury claims by year reported. We see here a clear growth in the number of injury claims made[1]. In 1989 well over twice as many claims were made compared with 1984[2]. The year 1987 constitutes an exception to this trend; for the slight drop in this particular year no explanation has been found. But this is *not* the case where the relatively large increase in the number of injury claims in 1988 is concerned. This increase is accounted for by one major incident which led to in-

Trend in injury claims submitted
N=1550

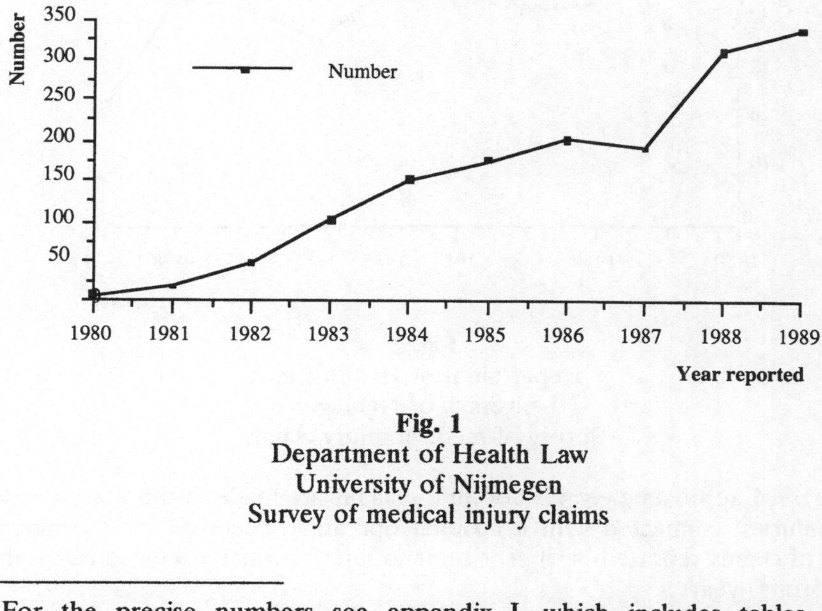

Fig. 1
Department of Health Law
University of Nijmegen
Survey of medical injury claims

---

[1] For the precise numbers see appendix I, which includes tables. The reference is as follows: Table 1.

[2] Since relatively few claims were made between 1980-1983, 1984 is generally taken as the first measuring point.

juries being suffered by a large number of patients, and more than 50 claims being made as a result. This justifies a correction to the year 1988.

When considering these figures, it must be borne in mind that a significant number of them "lag behind", by which is meant a situation in which a claim is, more often than not, not reported in the year during which the injury occurs (insurance companies use the term IBNR - Incurred But Not Reported - to cover this phenomenon). The survey reveals that injury claims are even not reported until 10 years after the injuries have occurred (Table 2)[3].

Trend in indemnities to patients
N=1549

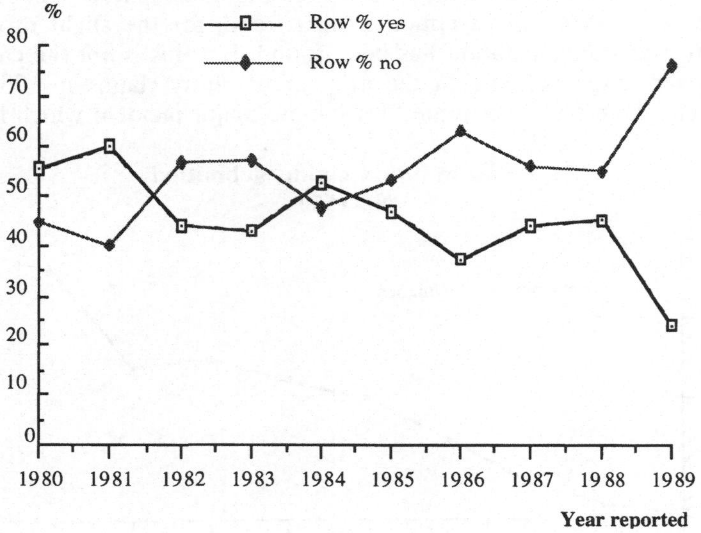

Fig. 2
Department of Health Law
University of Nijmegen
Survey of medical injury claims

Since 1984 approximately 40% of injury claims are made in the year in which the injuries, connected with a hospital operation, occurred. The remaining 60% of claims reported each year refer to injuries which occurred *before* that (reporting) year.

---

[3] Table 2 relates to 1538 injury claims. The remaining 12 cases in injury occurred *before* 1980. Accordingly, they are omitted.

The period covered by our survey is too limited to permit any more detailed pronouncements to be made about the pattern of IBNR's. But it is certainly to be expected that the number of claims relating to the survey period will continue to grow.
An interesting question here, of course, is what is happening with this clearly rising number of injury claims. In how many cases has an indemnity been paid during the period covered by the survey?

Down to the reference date an indemnity was paid in 626 cases (40%) (Table 3). Fig. 2 is a diagram showing the trend in the number of indemnities[4]. This shows that initially, in more than 50% of injury claims made, an indemnity has been paid. After this a gradual falling off begins. In 1984 we can see that the number of cases in which an indemnity is paid still predominates. After this point the lines clearly diverge and there is a proportionate fall in the number of cases in which the patient receives an indemnity. This fall becomes acute from 1988 onwards.

This fact is all the more significant because the claims cases involved in the random sample are overwhelmingly closed cases. The relatively limited number of unsettled cases here may, admittedly, bring about some change, but it must be taken into account that these unsettled cases are spread over a number of reporting years.
We have seen that the number of injury claims in which an indemnity is paid shows a relative fall. What is the trend in absolute terms in the number of injury claims in which an indemnity is paid?

The above bar chart provides some illustration on this point (fig. 3)[5]. It can be seen from this that the number of injury claims rises sharply, but that since 1984 the number of cases in which an indemnity is paid remains pretty much the same in absolute terms. Only 1988 represents something of a departure. Here, however, a correction may be made because, as remarked earlier, that particular year saw *one* incident which gave rise to several dozen claims. After this correction has been made we can see a more or less constant number of cases in which an indemnity was paid, viz. approximately 80 claims. This phenomenon naturally begs the question whether many claims are wrongly dismissed. In this connection we make the following observation.

---

[4] In the case of one claim it is not known whether any indemnity was awarded. This case has been omitted from our considerations.

[5] Here too, that claim in which it is not known whether an indemnity was paid, has been left out of consideration.

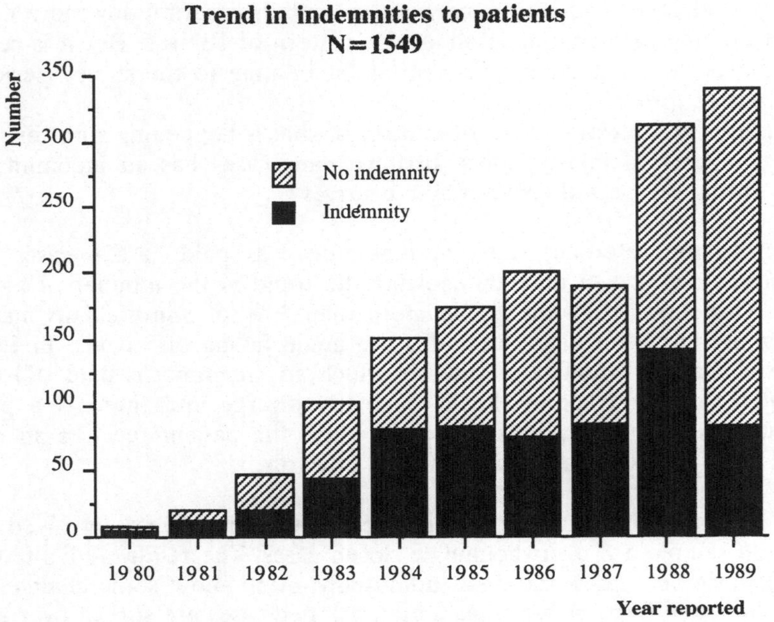

Fig. 3
Department of Health Law
University of Nijmegen
Survey of medical injury claims

A close study of those cases in which no indemnity was paid reveals the following picture (fig. 4). Out of a total of 552 closed cases in which the claim was dismissed, more than half of them end because the person submitting the claim takes no further action in response to the insurer's rejection (54%). In 16% of cases the person making the claim takes no further action after reporting the injury. In 6% of cases the claim has been withdrawn. In the category "other" (22.5%) we must assume that there has been acceptance of a dismissed claim following the advice of a neutral expert, no further action being taken following dismissal of a complaint by a medical disciplinary tribunal or by a medical inspector. It can also happen that an injury claim is not pursued after a medical disciplinary tribunal has upheld a complaint or following acknowledgment of liability by the insurer.

Table 4 in the Appendix provides a further breakdown of the methods of closure. The heading "More than one insurer" contains, *inter alia*, road traffic injuries for which liability exists on the basis of the Dutch Motor Vehicle Liability Insurance Act, an example of which is the case of a victim of a road traffic accident who is taken to hospital for the treatment of his injury and then experiences an injury as a result of incorrect medical treatment.

The category "other", for example, contains cases in which "no further action is taken after it is learned that the hospital has admitted liability" and also those cases in which the person concerned dies during settlement of the claim. This category also includes those cases in which the party involved has decided to let matters stand for the time being. It is generally the patient who makes this decision when it transpires that the extent of the injury is limited.

Manner of closing case: rejected claims
N=552

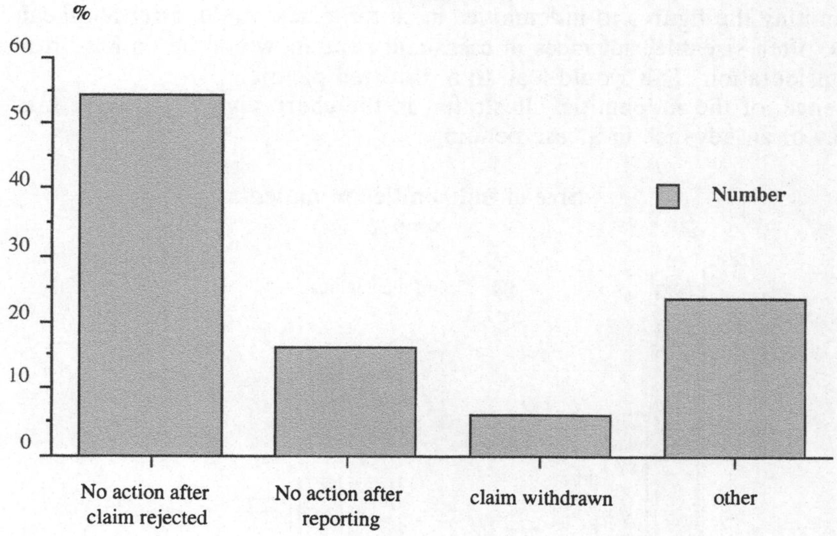

Fig. 4
Department of Health Law
University of Nijmegen
Survey of medical injury claims

The survey reveals that a good three quarters of the claims settled and dismissed end without any noticeable reaction on the part of the patient.

The patient evidently "quickly" accepts the situation when liability is repudiated. What could be the explanation for this state of affairs? Is the patient disinclined to take the long road of legal proceedings? Is he ignorant and lacking in expert legal assistance? Or is it simply the case that quite a lot of clearly unfounded claims are being made? This question cannot be answered, because an examination of the cases in which this is relevant furnishes no clarity in the matter.

What is the size of the indemnities paid during the period covered by the survey? The representative random sample gives the following picture, which is shown in the form of a bar chart (fig. 5). The data are given as percentages. Attention must be drawn to the fact that all these involve indemnities, which therefore include advances made in so called pending cases.

Furthermore, it must be said in passing that the advances made in pending cases during 1990 have also been incorporated in the chart. These advances have been included in the illustration to make it as complete as possible.

Limiting the figures to indemnities in closed cases would, after all, mean that all, often sizeable, advances in cases still pending would be omitted from the consideration. This would lead to a distorted picture.
Hence, of the indemnities illustrated in the chart, eighty (80) were made by way of an advance in a case pending.

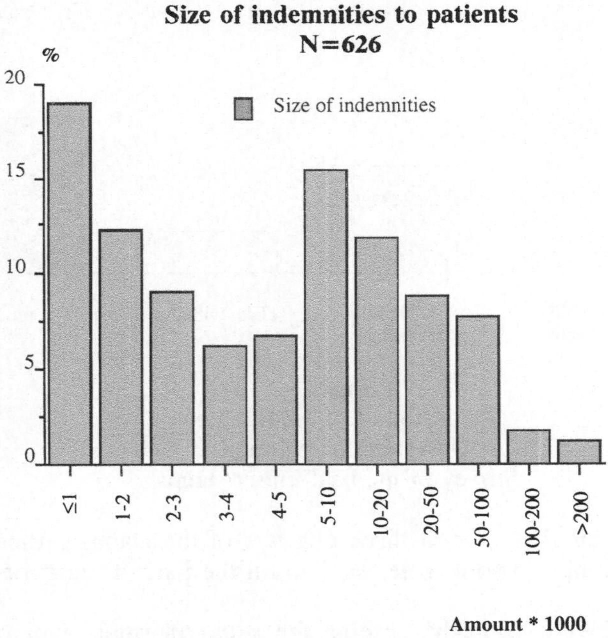

Fig. 5
Department of Health Law
University of Nijmegen
Survey of medical injury claims

We see here a concentration among the low indemnities. More than half of all indemnities are below ƒ 5,000.--. A good 15% of indemnities refer to an amount between ƒ 5,000.-- and ƒ 10,000.--. A good 10% of the indemnities are above ƒ 50,000.--, whilst in 3% of cases the indemnity is in excess of ƒ 100,000.-- (Table 5).

Attention is also drawn to claims in which an amount of ƒ 100,000.-- or more has been paid (Table 6). There are 20 of these. The table looks at how large the indemnities are and what the ratio is of compensation for property damage to compensation for pain and suffering. According to Table 6, two indemnities of ƒ 100,000.-- have been paid. The largest comes to ƒ 752,500.--. Of these claims 15 had been settled by the reference date, and 5 were still outstanding. In only one of these last mentioned cases can the possibility not be excluded that an indemnity will be paid to the patient.

Moreover, Table 6 shows that the compensation for pain and suffering differs greatly in the cases in question. The average amount paid for pain and suffering in percentage terms comes to 31.6%. A closer examination of the claims indemnities of ƒ 100,000.-- or above reveals that the pain and suffering payments differ much less in absolute terms. In 12 cases a figure of between ƒ 50,000.-- and ƒ 100,000.-- was paid for pain and suffering. In 3 of these cases the figure was between ƒ 15,000.-- and ƒ 30,000.--, while in one case the amount was approximately ƒ 8,000.--. In the remaining four cases it is not known how much was paid under this head[6].

Another question is whether, in the case of a number of indemnities which are approximately the same each year, the level of the indemnity rises sharply. The following bar chart (fig. 6) provides some insight into this. From this it will be seen that the number of large indemnities (over ƒ 50,000.--) does not increase during the period covered by the survey. We see that the large injury indemnities occur during a number of reporting years, including the early reporting years. For example, we find indemnities between ƒ 100,000.-- and ƒ 200,000.-- in the reporting years 1981, 1983, 1984, 1986 and 1987. The same picture is seen in the case of indemnities of over ƒ 200,000.-- (Table 7). A relatively sharp increase can be seen in the case of indemnities of up to ƒ 5,000.-- and in those of up to ƒ 10,000.--. On the basis of fig. 6 it can be stated that indemnities during the period covered by the survey, classified by the year in which the injury was reported, do not increase greatly in terms of amounts.

---

[6] Appendix II contains an overall description of these 20 claims. The review concludes with a brief commentary.

It is also interesting to look at the composition of these indemnities. What can we say about the compensation for pain and suffering?

Table 8 shows that in 470 claims there is compensation for pain and suffering (75% of indemnified claims). In almost 40% of injury claims honoured and involving pain and suffering, the level of the indemnity relating to this component remains unknown. This high percentage is to be explained by the fact that often a so called lump sum is paid to a patient. This means that a total sum in indemnification is paid out without any allocation to various indemnity items. Generally speaking, the indemnities mentioned here are exclusive of any reimbursement of costs in connection with a patient's legal assistance. Where lump sum indemnities are concerned this is not the case.

Trend in size of indemnities to patients
N=626

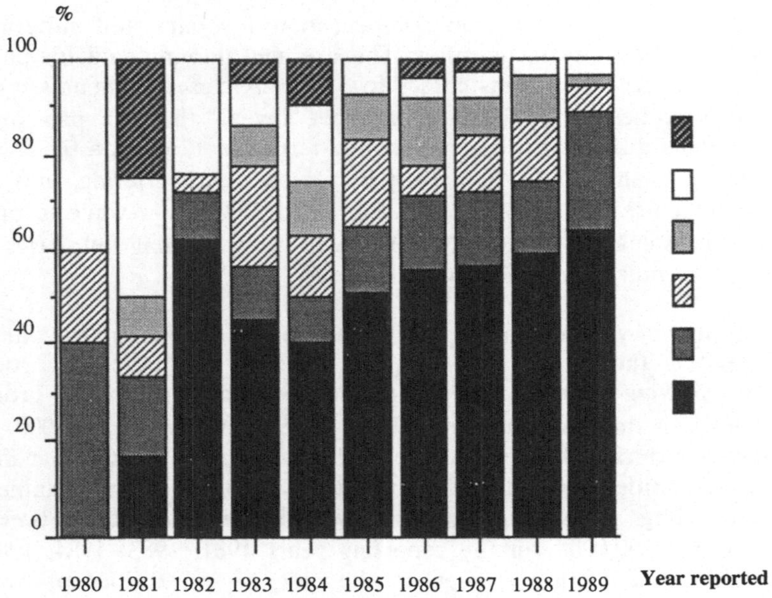

Fig. 6
Department of Health Law
University of Nijmegen
Survey of medical injury claims

Of those pain and suffering indemnities where the amount is known (n = 283) half is under a figure of *f* 5,000.00. A good 17% concerns a figure between *f* 5,000.-- and *f* 10,000.--, whilst in a good 5% there is a pain and suffering indemnity of from *f* 50,000.-- to *f* 100,000.--. There has, furthermore, been a statistical enquiry into whether there is any connection between the level of the total indemnity and the level of the pain and suffering indemnity, insofar as this is known. The result is a pretty high correlation at n = 283 (r = 0.64). This means that, as the total indemnity rises, so also does the payment for pain and suffering. If the pain and suffering component of the indemnity, insofar as this is known, is set against the total indemnity to the patient in these cases (n = 283) , the average pain and suffering indemnity turns out to be *f* 12,179.-- and the average total indemnity *f* 30,493.--. Moreover, the median indemnity is *f* 5,000.-- as against *f* 8,500.--, whilst the modal indemnity amounts to *f* 3,000.--, as against *f* 4,000.--. The survey reveals that in these cases the compensation for pain and suffering amounts on average to 43% of the total indemnity to the patient.

When an injury claim is made, it is of great importance to the insurer to discover as soon as possible the extent of the loss which has occurred. After the financial extent of the matter has been estimated on the basis of the data in the claims file, a sum is reserved corresponding to the expected (maximum) claim indemnity. If, during the course of the handling of the case, it transpires that the claim is turning out differently from what was initially expected, the level of the reserve is adjusted. Using these reserves, it is possible to construct a picture of the loss which will probably lead to an indemnity. In this way the insurer can form an idea of the anticipated total claims burden during a particular period, which is important for the conduct of his business.
An interesting question is the extent to which the abovementioned reserve method can be used as a means of forecasting the loss to be expected in pending cases. To this end the authors investigated what correlation exists between the reserves and the indemnities paid in cases already settled. Is it the case that the level of the reserve more or less corresponds to the actual indemnity or do both amounts differ sharply?

Of the 466 claims[7] it is the case that in 47 there is a reserve which is lower than the indemnity (10%). Furthermore, in 122 cases the reserve corresponds to the indemnity (26%)[8]. Moreover, in 91 cases the reserve turns out

---

[7] It was revealed earlier that out of the 626 indemnities, 546 had been paid in closed cases. Of these cases 80 have been disregarded in the attempt to answer the question about the relationship between the level of the reserve and the indemnity because in these cases the level of the reserve is not known.

[8] This category also includes those cases in which the reserve differs, either upwards or downwards, by more than 25% of the indemnity.

to be 125% to 200% of the indemnity (19.5%). In 127 cases the reserve is 2 to 5 times as large as the amount paid out as indemnity (27.3%), while in 46 cases the reserve is 5 to 10 times greater than the indemnity (9.8%). In addition, in 26 cases the reserve is 10 to 25 times greater than the indemnity paid (5.5%) and in 7 cases the reserve is seen to be more than 25 times the size of the indemnity (1.5%) (Table 9). In these 466 claims, there is a total reserve of *f* 13,604,300.--, whilst *f* 9,308,399.-- has been paid out as indemnity. In the cases in question an average sum of *f* 29,194.-- has been set aside as reserve and a figure of *f* 19,975.-- paid as an indemnity. If we confine ourselves to those cases in which a greater sum has been reserved than paid as indemnity (n = 353), we find that an average of *f* 17,311.-- more has been set aside as reserve than paid as an indemnity[9].

On the basis of the foregoing it can be established that the level of the reserves differs considerably from the level of indemnities. In this connection we must point out that it is noticeable that in creating the reserve the insurer also takes account of external costs, e.g. costs incurred for expert reports and the costs of the insurer's own legal advice. It is most probable that the insurer applies a fixed percentage to these. In insurance circles a figure of approximately 5% to cover these external costs is current.
Whatever the figure, these external costs cannot in any event provide an explanation for the fact that in general the amount paid out as an indemnity is two thirds of the sum applied as a reserve.

To summarise, it may be said, on the basis of the survey of closed cases, that the relationship between reserve and indemnity is too weak to allow it to be used in cases pending as a basis for predicting the expected indemnity.

---

[9] The connection between reserve and indemnity has also been calculated statistically for the 466 closed cases. This produces a correlation factor of .60. This means that in general there exists a fairly high correlation between indemnity and reserve. Further data reveal, incidentally, that in the case of indemnities of between *f* 20,000.-- and *f* 200,000.-- there exists a fairly high correlation (n=92). In the category "indemnities above *f* 200,000.--" (n=4) there is a negative correlation.

Chapter 3

INJURY CLAIMS AND PROCEDURES

Liability at civil law for medical acts may be based on an attributable failure pursuant to Art. 6:74 Dutch Civil Code and/or an unlawful act pursuant to Art. 6:162 Dutch Civil Code. The first case involves a failure on the part of a professional practitioner in the discharge of his contractual obligations. The second possibility concerns an extra-contractual liability.

It is not always clear from the claims investigated which alternative has been chosen as a basis. In most cases the basis on which liability is attributed is not, or is hardly ever, cited. Moreover, it cannot be discerned from the available material whether it is solely the person(s) rendering medical assistance who has/have been held liable or whether the institution in which the accident occurred has also been held liable for the injury. These data are usually absent in the claims file.

In how many cases is liability admitted by the insurer? The survey reveals that in 32% of indemnity cases liability for the medical act/treatment is admitted. In 43.5% of cases liability is repudiated, while in the remaining 24% of cases the position is not known. This last mentioned figure can also mean that the insurer has not yet taken a position (Table 10).

We have already seen that in some 40% of cases in the survey an indemnity has been paid. In view of the fact that liability is admitted in only 32% of cases, we may infer that not every indemnity is based upon an admission of liability. This category of indemnities may include cases in which no position regarding liability is known and sometimes where liability has been repudiated. In this last case we speak of "accommodation payments".

The purpose of the survey was not to deal with the question of whether the repudiation of a particular injury claim was right or not. Yet it is worth noting one or two points here. It is to be expected that injury claims which have been wrongly repudiated by insurers will lead to action being taken elsewhere. Civil actions, complaints to medical disciplinary tribunals and to the medical inspectorate of the Health Service spring to mind. The survey looked at whether the steep increase in the number of rejected claims during the survey period had led to more actions being brought and complaints being made elsewhere.

The diagram below (fig. 7)[1] makes clear that during the period covered by the survey there was no increase in the number of civil actions arising from claims submitted. Even more striking is the fact that the number of civil actions has actually fallen (Table 11). This confirms, incidentally, the expectation that, with regard to medical injury claims, civil actions are begun only in very few cases, viz. approximately 4% (63)[2]. For the sake of completeness it is worth noting that some of the outstanding cases may perhaps still lead to the initiation of civil proceedings[3]. Where the relevant civil actions are concerned, it also transpires that in 41% of disputes referred to the courts, including those in which it is the level of the indemnity which is being contested, the actions are successful.

Trend in civil actions
N=1548

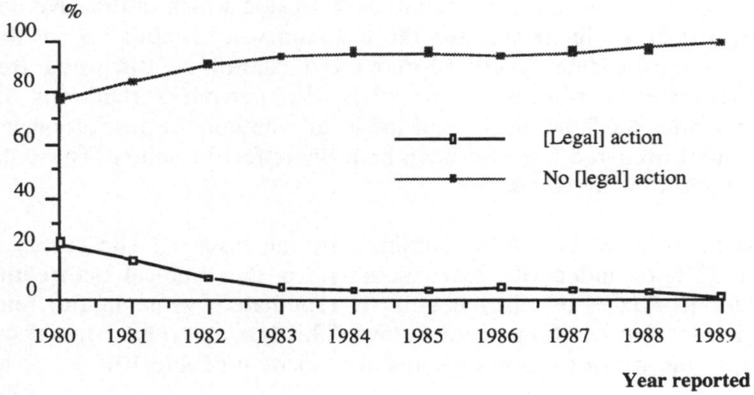

Fig. 7
Department of Health Law
University of Nijmegen
Survey of medical injury claims

---

[1] In 2 cases it is not known whether a civil action was brought. These cases have been disregarded here.

[2] J.H. Hubben, The Civil Courts and Medical Injury claims. In: Grenzen aan de zorg; zorgen aan de grens, Alphen a/d Rijn, 1990, pp. 205-220.

[3] Of 37 civil actions in which the claim was not allowed, 29 cases are still being dealt with on the reference date. Based on an average indemnity percentage (40%), this means that in approximately 12 cases an indemnity may be expected.

If we look at the level of indemnities in cases in which a civil action has been brought (n = 26), we find the following: the average indemnity is *f* 107,509.-, the median *f* 25,356.- and the modus *f* 10,000.-. For purposes of comparison we give below the abovementioned values with reference to that group of indemnities in cases in which no civil action has been brought (n = 599). Here the average indemnity comes to *f* 16,052.-, the median value being *f* 4,700.-, while the modus is *f* 5,000.-.

The question arises as to what significance should be attached to the considerable difference in indemnities with and without the intervention of the civil courts. Obviously we may assume that the issues involved in cases relating to medical injury brought before the courts are much more serious and therefore lead to larger indemnities.

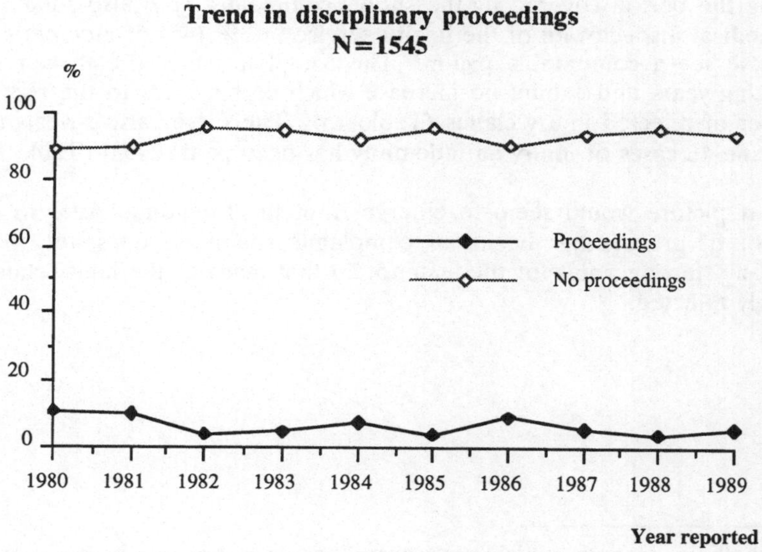

Fig. 8
Department of Health Law
University of Nijmegen
Survey of medical injury claims

The survey also examines in how many cases an action has been brought before a medical disciplinary tribunal (fig. 8)[4]. During the period under review this proves to be so in 6% of cases (n = 92). In examining the distribution of

[4] In 5 cases it is not known whether a complaint was made to a medical disciplinary tribunal. These cases have been disregarded in the survey.

figures over the years covered by the survey we detect no increase in the number of disciplinary procedures to match the rise in the number of repudiated claims (Table 12). The number of complaints upheld by medical disciplinary tribunals corresponds to 25% (Table 13)[5], a percentage which, by the way, does not differ noticeably from the number of complaints (in percentage terms) generally upheld over the years by medical disciplinary tribunals.

It transpires, incidentally, that in 21% of injury claims in which disciplinary proceedings were brought an indemnity was also paid (Table 14)[6]. It is likewise appropriate to note that in some of the cases in which a complaint has been made to a medical disciplinary tribunal and which are outstanding, indemnities may still be expected.

During the period covered by the survey complaints were also submitted to the medical inspectorate of the health service in 3% (46) of indemnity cases. Here we see a comparable picture. The complaints are spread over all the reporting years and exhibit no increase which corresponds to the rise in the number of rejected injury claims (Table 15)[7]. The survey also reveals that in 11 of the 46 cases of injury an indemnity has been paid (24%) (Table 16)[8].

A clear picture would seem to emerge from the foregoing. Analysis of the number of proceedings begun or complaints submitted does not, in itself, offer any starting point for the assumption that many of the injury claims are wrongly rejected.

---

5 Both those cases in which no proceedings were brought before a medical disciplinary tribunal (1453) and those in which it is not known whether a disciplinary complaint was made are included here as "missing cases".

6 There are 5 cases in which it is not known whether medical disciplinary tribunal proceedings were initiated. These cases have been omitted from the survey.

7 In 3 cases it is not known whether a complaint was submitted to the medical inspectorate. These cases have been omitted.

8 In 3 cases it is not known whether a complaint was submitted to the medical inspectorate, while in one of these cases it is also not known whether an indemnity was paid. These 3 cases have been omitted.

In only 10 cases were both civil law and disciplinary tribunal proceedings begun (Table 17)[9].

Of the 10 cases in which both civil law and disciplinary tribunal proceedings were initiated there were 4 closed cases and 6 still being dealt with on the reference date. Of the 4 closed cases an indemnity had been paid in two of them (both around the *f* 20,000.-- figure).

In the 2 other cases which had been settled and in which no indemnity had been paid, both the complaint to the medical disciplinary tribunal and the civil law claim had been dismissed.

As far as concerns current claims (6) it is the case that in 4 of these the complaint to the disciplinary tribunal was (eventually) upheld, in one the complaint was dismissed and in the other one no decision had been announced by the reference date. In 2 cases in which the complaint was upheld the claim at civil law had also partly succeeded. In both cases advances had been paid by the reference date, these being to the value of *f* 100,000.-- and *f* 80,000.--. In the 2 other cases in which the claim was upheld, the civil courts gave an interlocutory judgment in one case, while in the other judgment was reserved in order that composition proposals might be made.

In the current case in which the disciplinary tribunal complaint was dismissed, the judge in the civil proceedings called for an expert's report. No payment had (yet) been made on the reference date for this case. In the last of the 6 current cases both the disciplinary complaint and the civil law claim were still being heard on the reference date.

Closely connected with the question of the procedures employed is that of the manner of legal assistance. The survey reveals that in 60% of the injury claims investigated there was some form of legal aid (Table 18)[10]. Where legal assistance was provided, in 73% of cases this was given by an attorney at law. The large category "other" consists of legal assistance provided by the ombudsman, consumer associations, recourse agencies, insurance agents. This category also includes those cases in which several parties have been involved

---

[9] There are 5 cases in which it is not known whether medical disciplinary proceedings were begun. Moreover, there are 2 cases, in which it is not known whether a civil law action was begun. One case, incidentally, falls into both categories. These cases, 6 in all, have been omitted from our considerations here.

[10] In 8 cases it is not known whether there was legal assistance; these cases have not been considered here.

in providing legal assistance, e.g. when the person making an injury claim has changed his lawyer or when both a lawyer and a claims settlement agency are involved. Incidentally, it is important to note that the Table also includes those cases in which a third party submits an injury claim and those cases in which there is no injury claim.

Trend in provision of legal assistance to patients
N=1542

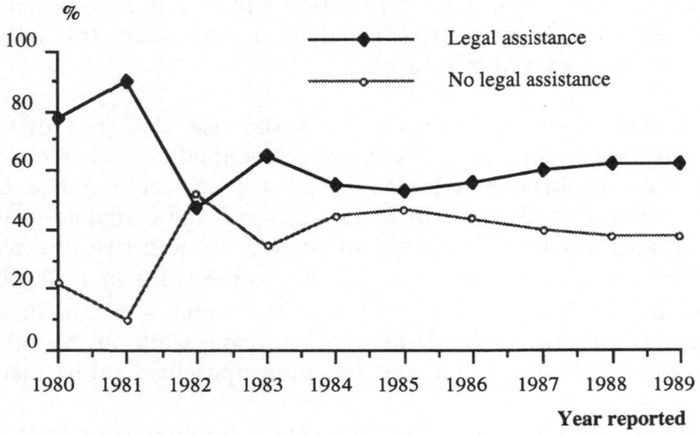

Fig. 9
Department of Health Law
University of Nijmegen
Survey of medical injury claims

Trends in legal assistance during the period covered by the survey were also examined. The above diagram (fig. 9) shows that in 1982 the percentage of cases with and without legal assistance was approximately the same. After this point in time we see the start of an increase in cases where there is legal assistance, rising to approximately 55% in 1984. Thereafter we see the percentage of cases with legal assistance rising slightly (Table 19)[11]. The graph does not show the fact that the decision of the Dutch Supreme Court dated 3rd April 1987, NJ 1988, 275, which laid down that the costs of legal assistance provided in connection with an injury claim also qualify for reimbursement, may have contributed to an increase in legal assistance.

Next, it is interesting to look at the effects of legal assistance being employed. Generally speaking, it can be said that legal assistance has a positive effect on the level of indemnities.

---

[11] *Vide* note 23.

If we regard the injury claims in Table 20[12], in which an indemnity has been paid after legal assistance has been enlisted, as the first group (n = 381), and those injury claims in which an indemnity was paid without the enlistment of legal assistance as the second group (n = 244), the difference in the level of the indemnities paid between the two groups becomes significant (t=0.00 at a 5% level). In group 1 the average indemnity is ƒ 29,501.--, while in group 2 it is ƒ 4,576.--. This means that in indemnity cases in which there has been legal assistance, on average almost six times more is paid out (to the patient). The median value in group 1 is ƒ 9,000.-- and the modal indemnity comes to ƒ 5,000.--, whereas in group 2 the median is ƒ 1,626.-- and the modal indemnity ƒ 2,000.--.

Some qualification is not out of place here because it is plausible that in the case of minor damage or injury as a result of correct/incorrect procedure in a hospital, a patient is more likely to look after his own interests, whereas in the case of serious damage or injury it is more likely that legal assistance will be enlisted. As a result of this effect, the level of indemnities up to ƒ 5,000.-- is comparable for both groups. Here too, one may speak of a significant difference (t=0.00 at a 5% level). In group 1 the average indemnity is ƒ 2,849.--, while in group 2 the average is ƒ 1,543.--.

Where relatively low indemnities are concerned, it would, therefore, appear that in cases in which use is made of legal assistance the average indemnity is almost twice as high.

In addition to the method of legal assistance, the authors also looked at the extent to which medical assistance plays a role in the settlement of medical injury claims. Such assistance is generally afforded by a neutral expert physician, who draws up a report. As a rule this person plays an important role in the settlement of an indemnity claim. It is plausible to suggest that where such a person is required to state an opinion concerning the culpability of the person who performed the operation by investigating either whether the treatment was incorrect or careless or whether any causal connection exists between the incorrect action and the injury sustained, this opinion will be accepted by the insurers.

The survey shows (Table 21) that in 388 cases a neutral expert physician was enlisted (25%). It is striking that in only 4% of these cases a neutral expert opinion is issued at the patient's initiative. In the overwhelming number of

---

[12] There are 8 cases in which it is not known whether an indemnity was enlisted. Moreover, in one of these cases it is also not known whether an indemnity was paid. These cases are omitted from our considerations here.

cases the neutral expert physician is chosen by mutual consultation (between the patient and the insurer).

The survey then goes on to look at the task of the neutral expert physician (Table 22)[13]. The purpose of the majority of opinions - insofar as this can be deduced from the claims files - is to answer the question whether there has been a case of careless/incorrect act and whether there is a (sufficient) causal connection between the incorrect act and the injury sustained (67%; n = 358).

In 17% of cases the neutral expert was asked to give an opinion on the degree of a patient's permanent disability as a result of an incorrect procedure. Only in 14% of these opinions has a pronouncement been made on both the question of whether good medical practice has been employed and/or whether there is any causal connection and on the extent of disability.

The survey additionally reveals that it is rare for a second neutral expert to be enlisted. There are only 49 cases (approximately 3%) (Table 23). In the cases relevant here what we have, for example, is a neutral expert whose terms of reference are to establish the degree of permanent disability, after a different expert has been asked at an earlier stage to assess the degree of care exercised by the operator involved in the incident.

It also happens that the opinion of the neutral expert physician does not agree with the viewpoint of the patient (or of the person defending his/her interests). In such cases it is always possible to seek an opinion from another expert. This is seldom if ever done by the patient. This fact, too, leads one to suspect that the person submitting an injury claim is not always capable of reacting adequately when the insurer rejects a claim: on this point see also the note in Table 4.

In addition to legal assistance the survey also examined a number of other aspects relating to the patient.

First of all the person submitting the claim was considered. The survey reveals that in 80% of cases it is the patient himself who takes the initiative and submits a claim for damages for the injury he has suffered in connection with the medical treatment he has undergone (Table 24)[14]. In 4% of cases it

[13] In 30 cases in which a neutral expert physician was involved, his task is not known. These cases have been omitted.

[14] In 58 cases it is not known who the claimant is. These cases have been disregarded.

is the family which takes the initiative; this category includes the patient's spouse and children.
The category "others" (1%) is formed by third parties, e.g. sickness fund, employer, trade union. We are talking here only about cases in which third parties submit a claim in respect of a medical operation on a specified person. In these cases the patient himself claims nothing.
In nearly 3% of cases there was no claimant. In the strict sense of the word no claim arises in these cases. What we are concerned with here is so called *pro forma* reports by (usually) the hospital in its capacity of insured party. The insured informs the insurance company that an accident has occurred. Because these cases can be regarded as potential claims, they have been included in the survey.
In addition, there are cases in which both the patient and a third party submit a claim to obtain indemnification of a loss as a result of a medical act/treatment in the hospital. In 6% of the cases investigated a claim has (also) been made by a third party (n = 90). The vast majority of these cases concern a claim by the sickness costs insurer (including the sickness fund) in connection with sickness costs which have been reimbursed to the hospital (Table 25). The category "other" includes the Motor Vehicle Liability Insurer; here one may be put in mind of a situation involving a road traffic accident *and* a medically incorrect treatment. Moreover, this category also includes cases in which more than one third party has submitted a claim, e.g. employer *and* sickness fund. Furthermore, it transpires that rather more than a half of the claims made by third parties succeed, viz. 57%. In the remaining cases either the claim is dismissed or we do not know what becomes of it (Table 26).

The majority of indemnities (65%) are below *f* 10,000.--. If we compare indemnities to third parties with those to patient, family or relatives, we see that the percentage of awards is somewhat higher (57% compared with 40%). The median, too, is greater where indemnities to third parties are concerned than in the case of indemnities to patients, viz. *f* 6,000.-- as against *f* 5,000.--. On the other hand, the average indemnity is appreciably lower, viz. *f* 5,396.-- as against *f* 19,825.--.

How do patients who have submitted an injury claim break down on the basis of sex?
If we look at the composition of the Netherlands population in terms of sex, we see that the ratio is 50:50% (Central Bureau of Statistics Year Book 1991). The survey reveals that 60% of patients are females and 40% male (Table 27)[15].

---

[15] In 7 cases the sex of the claimant is not known. These cases have been disregarded.

That more women, relatively speaking, submit claims can be explained by the fact that women make a greater claim on the health service. This can be seen from the bar charts below, which have been taken from the report Choosing and Sharing - Principal Recommendations of the Dunning Commission 1992. Fig. 10 shows that particularly where psychiatric disorders are concerned and in the case of motor disorders women make a greater claim on the health service.

Costs of care by disorder

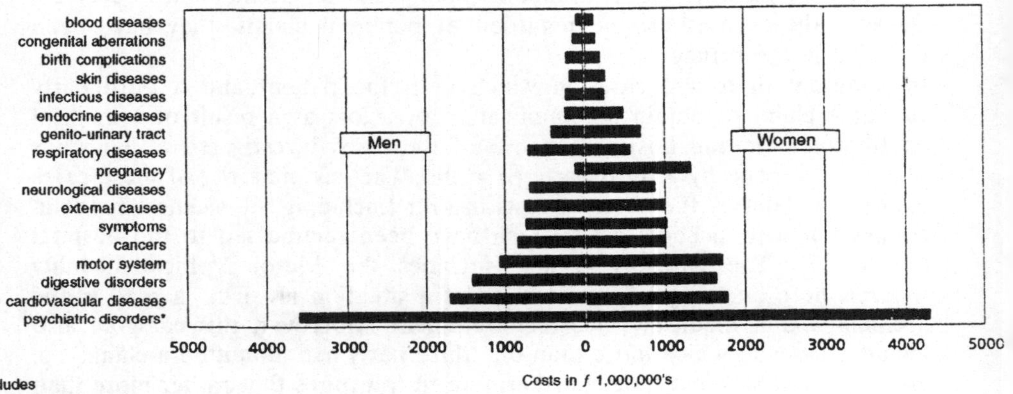

*includes mental deficiency and dementia

Source: Institute for Social Public health, Erasmus University Rotterdam

Fig. 10

Department of Health Law
University of Nijmegen
Survey of medical injury claims

If we consider the age composition of Dutch patients, it emerges that as age rises the consumption of public health facilities rises too (fig. 11).
The age distribution in our survey does not agree with this general picture (Table 28)[16]. The most striking fact is that, proportionally, elderly patients (> 71 years) submit few claims. Moreover, the average age of claimants turns out to be 40. The median, too, is 40. The age at which most indemnity claims occur (51) is from 0 to 1 year (modus).
If we look at the indemnity/no indemnity ratio, it emerges that in the case of women (n = 928) 46% of claims are met, whereas in the case of men (n = 614) 32% are accepted. It follows from this that, relatively speaking,

[16] In 133 cases the age is not known. These cases have been disregarded.

more injury claims from women are accepted than from men (Table 29)[17]. It also emerges from further data that the median value in relation to the level of the indemnity is the same for both sexes, viz. *f* 5,000.--. On the other hand, the level of the average indemnity in both groups does not agree; the average indemnity paid to male patients is *f* 28,100.--, while an average figure of *f* 16,100.-- is paid to females. This difference is significant at a 5% level (t=0.00 at a 5% level).

Costs per person in *f* 1,000's

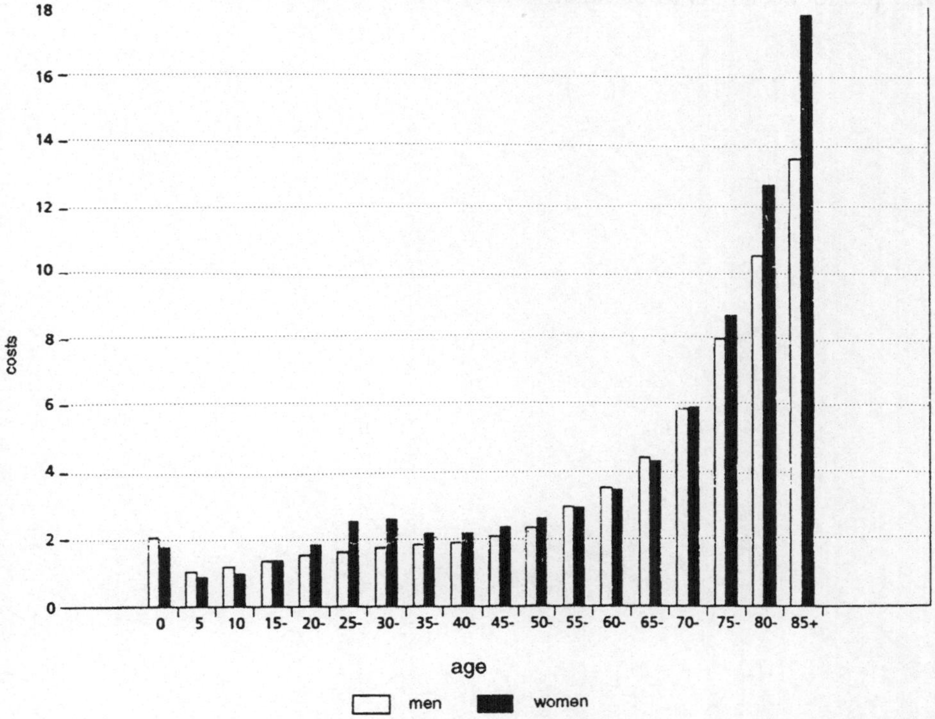

Fig. 11
Department of Health Law
University of Nijmegen
Survey of medical injury claims

---

[17] In 7 cases the sex of the person submitting the injury claim is not known and in 1 case it is not known whether an indemnity was paid or not. These cases have been omitted.

We see, therefore, that a higher indemnity is more often paid to men than to women. The reason for this is presumably to be found in the fact that men more often receive income from work than women. The financial consequences of an incorrect medical act are, as a result, more clearly visible and measurable.

The survey also reveals that a record of the patient's profession/occupation is only made on an incidental basis. Only in 27% of all cases do we know anything about the patient's profession/occupation, which is too little to allow any pronouncements to be made (Table 30).

Chapter 4

MEDICAL ASPECTS OF THE CLAIM

We now turn our attention to a number of medical aspects of an injury claim. The vast majority of claims (approximately 75%) relate to medical operations in a general hospital. A further statistic is that 22% of claims are made against university hospitals (Table 31)[1]. The category "other hospitals" includes rehabilitation centres and maternity hospitals.

Apart from this, the survey also reveals that the percentage of claims accepted in respect of university hospitals is higher than in general hospitals (45% as against 39%) (Table 32)[2].

To what medical operations do injury claims refer? The bar chart below (fig. 12) sheds some light on this (Table 33). This classification makes use of the Standard Classification for Specialist Medical Operations[3].

The lion's share of injury claims relates to surgical operations (44%)[4]. Diagnostic procedures account for approximately 19%, while 26% of injury claims relate to a category described as "other therapeutic procedures". This last named category includes anaesthetics, the application of dressings, splints and plaster casts, and also PTCA[5], *in vitro* fertilisation or laser therapy. The category "other" does not refer to medical operations, but concerns nursing

---

1 In 4 injury claims the type of hospital is not known. These cases have been disregarded.

2 In 4 injury claims the type of hospital is not known and in 1 case it is not clear whether or not an indemnity was paid. These 5 cases are not included here.

3 National Council of Public Health, Zoetermeer, 1990; 2nd ed.

4 Broadly speaking the category "surgical procedures" includes all procedures involving an incision (laparoscopy, arthroscopy etc.). Diagnostic procedures include all X-ray procedures, and also viewing procedures not involving an incision (e.g. bronchoscopy, angiography etc.).

5 Percutaneous transluminase coronary angioplasty

or care and attendance. In one single case the injury claim related to the fact that no treatment at all was given, for example, the patient was not admitted to hospital, even though, according to the patient, this was indicated.

Classification of medical operations
N=1550

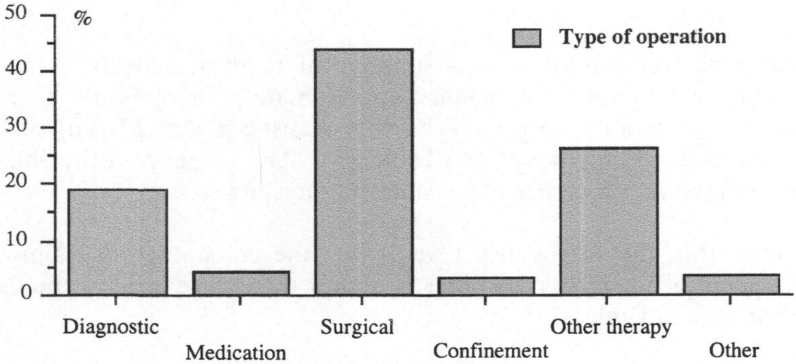

Fig. 12
Department of Health Law
University of Nijmegen
Survey of medical injury claims

An interesting question is whether the chance of an indemnity differs according to the different types of operation. Table 34[6] shows that, particularly in the case of medication (51%), confinement (49%) and "other therapeutic procedures" (48%), indemnities are, relatively speaking, paid frequently. In terms of indemnity percentages, surgical and diagnostic procedures do not differ greatly from one another (38% and 35% respectively).

We have seen that the 2 largest categories of procedure are operations and other therapeutic procedures. Table 35 breaks down these surgical procedures according to the Standard Classification. The survey included 680 cases of surgical procedure (44%). The largest group of claims relating to surgical procedures concerns operations to the musculo-skeletal system (29%).

We mentioned earlier that women make a greater claim on public health than men, a phenomenon which also finds its expression in the fact that almost 18% of the operations in respect of which a claim has been made relate to operations to the female genitalia or breasts. In contrast to this is

[6] The claim in which it is not known whether or not an indemnity was paid has been disregarded here.

the fact that surgical procedures on male sexual organs account for only 3%. Another category of operations which often, relatively speaking, leads to claims being made is that which concerns the digestive tract (gastro-intestinal operations) (10%).

The category "other therapeutic procedures" contains 406 injury claims (Table 36). The largest group of procedures in this category in respect of which claims have been submitted is formed by anaesthetics (38%). We have noted earlier that the category "other" procedures (27%) includes PTCA, dental treatment other than extractions (this last procedure is classified under oral cavity procedures), injections, phototherapy, physiotherapy etc. In addition, 14% of cases relate to dressings, splints and reductions.

Operator
N=1497

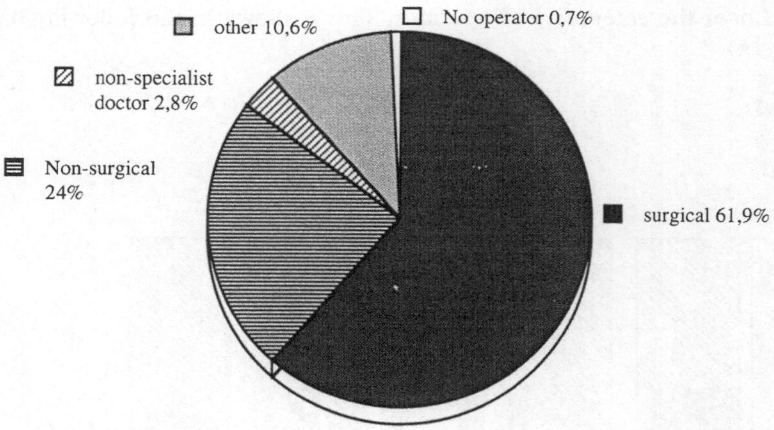

Fig. 13
Department of Health Law
University of Nijmegen
Survey of medical injury claims

If we look next at those persons performing the procedures to which the claims refer (fig. 13)[7], we find that 62% of injury claims concern a surgeon. 24% of the cases involve a non-surgical specialist. The fairly large category "other" deserves a note in passing. In point of fact, this category embraces 2 groups, viz. analysts and nurses. The large number of analysts is misleading

---

[7] In 52 cases the person performing the operation is not known. These cases have not been included.

because this refers to the injury claim mentioned earlier in which one procedure by an analyst is associated with a large number of injury claims. We also see a small number (3%) of non-specialist doctors acting as operators.

Finally there is a category called "no operator", which covers incidents in which no operator is involved. These claims involve cases of patients falling over in toilets or showers or out of bed.

It should, incidentally, be pointed out that where these operators are concerned no pronouncements are being made about the culpability of the action of the person rendering the medical assistance nor, in a more general sense, about liability. It is simply intended to indicate in which particular specialist field the claim has arisen.

The next point of interest is to look at how the number of indemnities is distributed over the categories of operator. This is shown in the following bar chart (fig. 14).

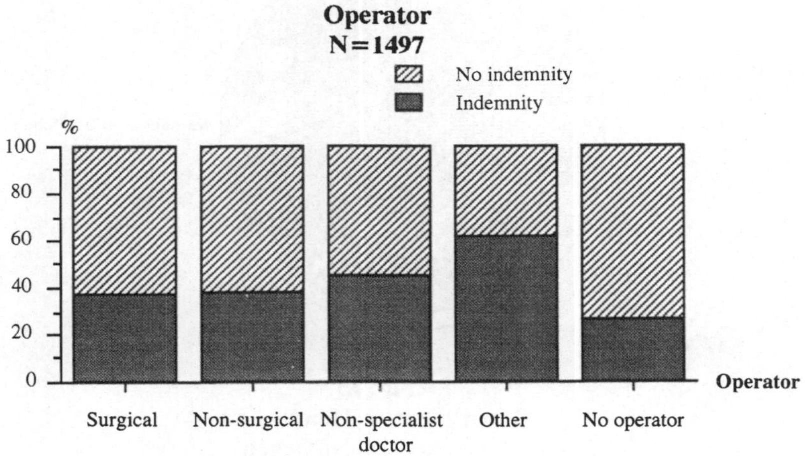

Fig. 14
Department of Health Law
University of Nijmegen
Survey of medical injury claims

This shows that, although the number of injury claims in the category "surgeons" is much larger than in the category "non-surgeons", the number of cases in which an indemnity is awarded is, proportionally, the same (Table

37)[8]. This raises questions about the basis of premium differentiation applied by insurers between surgeons and non-surgeons.

Are there indeed differences to be detected within that category of claims made against surgeons (fig. 15)[9]? Large groups within this category would appear to be general surgeons (33%), orthopaedic surgeons (16%), gynaecologists (17%) and oral surgeons (6%). The category "other" (28%) includes ENT specialists (6%), urologists (5.4%), plastic surgeons (3.6%) and ophthalmic surgeons (3.3%) (Table 38)[10].

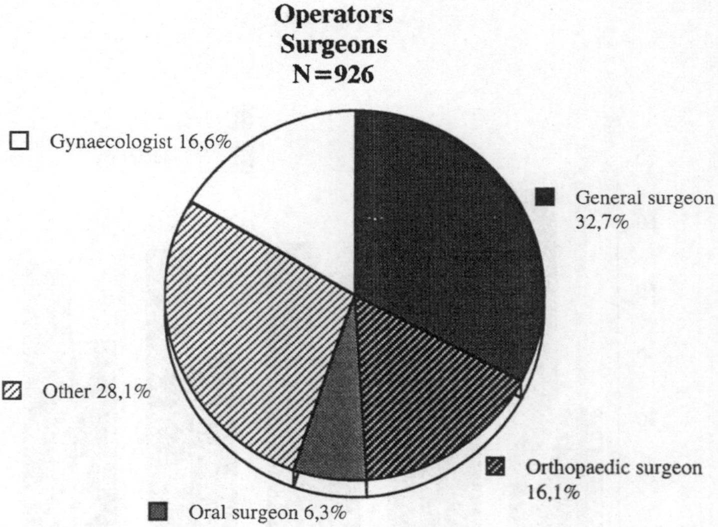

Fig. 15
Department of Health Law
University of Nijmegen
Survey of medical injury claims

---

8 In 52 cases the person performing the operation is not known. Also, in 1 case it is not known whether an indemnity was paid. These cases have not been included.

9 Table 37 shows that the category "surgeons" relates to 926 injury claims (62%).

10 The claim in which it is not known whether or not an indemnity was paid has been disregarded here.

The following bar chart shows the percentage of injury claims made against 1 of the said categories of surgeons, in which an indemnity was paid (fig. 16). During the period covered by the survey more indemnities were awarded, in percentage terms, for claims against gynaecologists (44%) and oral surgeons (41%) than against general surgeons and orthopaedic surgeons.

In these last named categories the number of cases in which an indemnity was paid was 33% and 36% respectively.

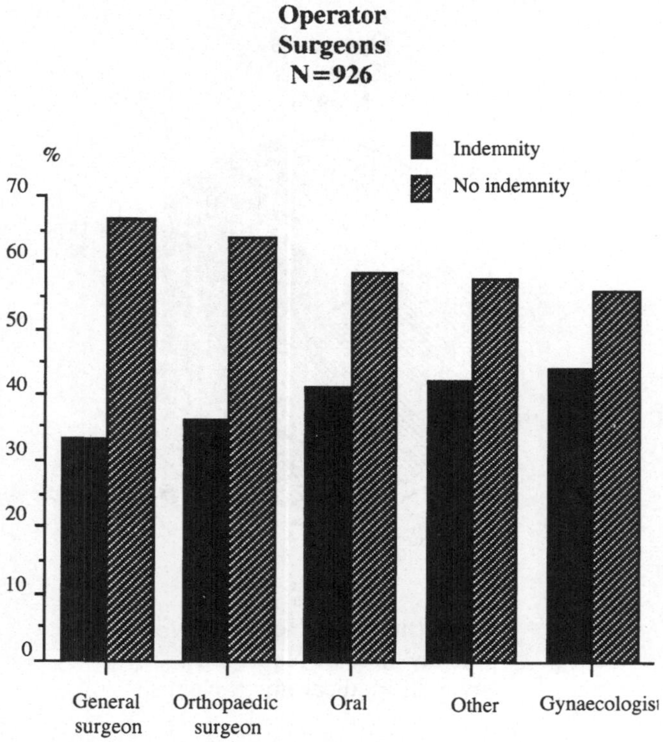

Fig. 16
Department of Health Law
University of Nijmegen
Survey of medical injury claims

In the category of injury claims made against non-surgical specialists (n = 360) which, as we have seen, is much smaller than the category "surgeons", we find from the pie chart below (fig. 17) that about half the injury claims submitted relate to the actions of anaesthetists (51%). Next come relatively large groups, viz. specialists in internal disorders (14%), radiologists

(10%), neurologists (8%), while the category "other" (18%) is accounted for by, among others, cardiologists (4.7%), paediatricians (2.2%) and pulmonary specialists (1.9%) (Table 39). The large percentage of anaesthetists deserves an observation in passing. This may easily create the impression that a great many mistakes are made in the actual administering of anaesthetic. Many injury claims against anaesthetists, however, relate to mistakes in intubation, with the resulting dental lesions.

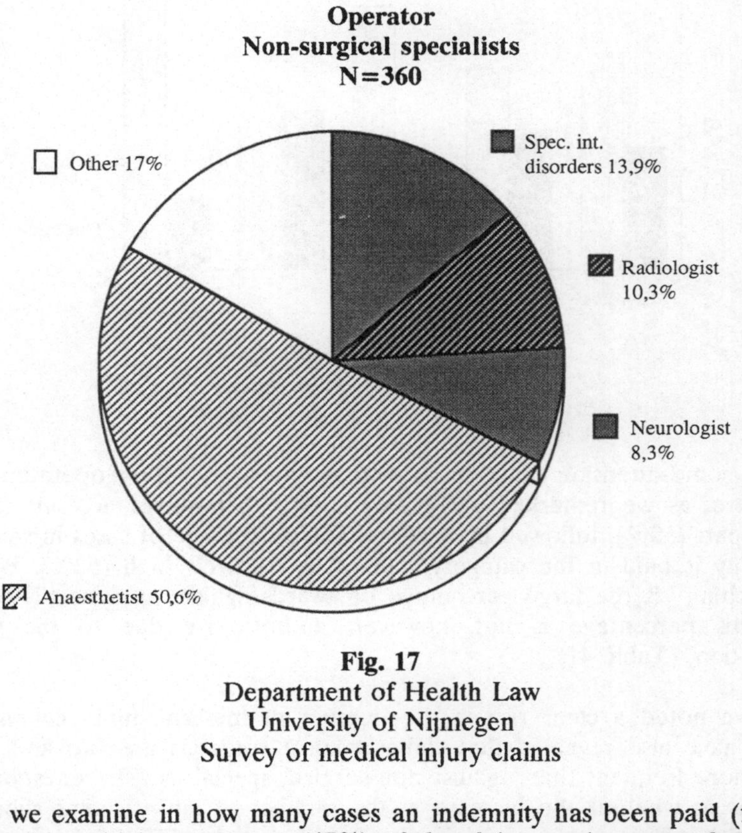

Fig. 17
Department of Health Law
University of Nijmegen
Survey of medical injury claims

When we examine in how many cases an indemnity has been paid (fig. 18), we see that a high percentage (47%) of the claims against anaesthetists are met. This percentage is lower for radiologists (41%), specialists in internal disorders (36%) and neurologists (23%).

With regard to the category "non-specialist doctors" the following may be said (Table 40). As far as concerns accident and emergency doctors, 40% of claims are accepted. In injury claims made against the acts of registrars, an indemnity is paid in 61.5% of cases.

Operator
Non-surgical specialists
N=360

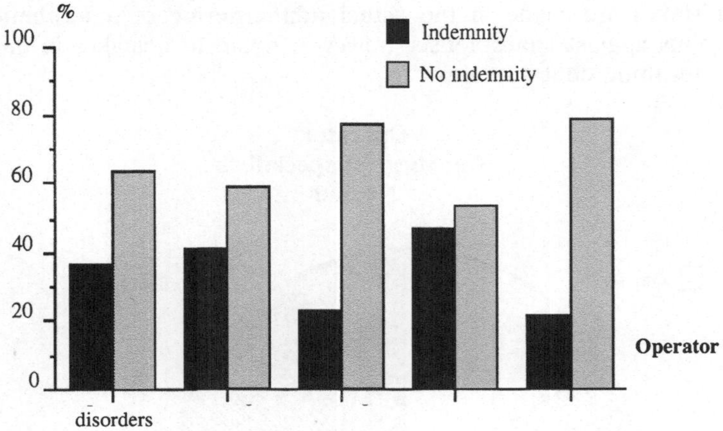

Fig. 18
Department of Health Law
University of Nijmegen
Survey of medical injury claims

Finally, some attention must be paid to the category "other operators" (fig. 19). Here, as we remarked earlier, we notice that nurses account for the largest part (50%), followed by analysts. The percentage of cases in which an indemnity is paid in the category "nurses" is relatively high (52%). What is eye-catching is the large percentage of awards against analysts (79%) (fig. 20). This percentage is not, however, authoritative due to the earlier explanation, (Table 41).

We have noted a clear rise in the number of medical injury claims. The figures have also revealed that claims against surgeons are two and a half times more frequent than against non-surgical specialists. The question now arises as to whether the increase in the number of injury claims submitted during the survey period is evenly distributed over the different categories of operator (Table 42)[11].

[11] As mentioned earlier, those cases in which the operator is not known (52) are left out of consideration.

Operator
Others
N=158

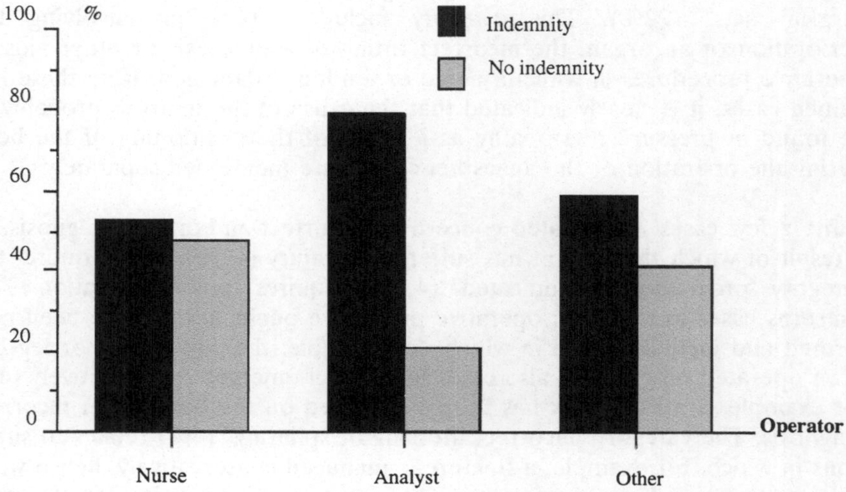

Fig. 19
Department of Health Law
University of Nijmegen
Survey of medical injury claims

The survey reveals that the share of the category "surgeons" increases steadily during the period covered by the survey (6% in 1984 to 14% in 1989)[12]. It can also be seen that the percentage of claims involving non-surgical specialists (n = 360) is fairly constant between 1984 and 1988 (2.7%; n = 1498). In the following years the percentage goes up to 6.7% in 1989.

Likewise, in the category "other operators" (n = 158) the percentage of claims between 1984 and 1988 remains fairly constant (approximately 1%; n = 1498). In 1988 this figure rises to 4.7%. The reason for this increase is to be found in the 54 IVF cases, in which an analyst was involved. In 1989 a fall in the claims percentage becomes noticeable.
Given the smallness of both categories, viz. "non-specialist doctors" and "no operator", no further consideration is given to them.
To summarise, it is apparent that the increase in the total number of claims occurs particularly in the category "surgeons".

[12] In this connection the grand total (1498) (Table 41) has been taken as the bases for arriving at percentages.

We saw earlier what medical procedures the injury claims relate to. It is of interest to note in what specific medical context the claim is submitted. What, according to the patient, has gone wrong from a medico-technical point of view (Table 43)[13]? The largest group of claims relates to "technico-surgical acts" (22%). This category includes operations involving the perforation of an organ, the incorrect fitting of a prothesis or other aids or operative procedures in which a nerve or tendon is damaged. If, in these last named cases, it is clearly indicated that the cause of the injury is probably to be found in pressure neuropathy as a result of the positioning of the body during the operation or the anaesthetic, they are mentioned separately.

Quite a few cases investigated concern an incorrect and/or late diagnosis, as a result of which the patient has suffered an injury (12%). Furthermore, the category "procedure not indicated" (4.5%) requires some explanation. This concerns cases in which an operative procedure ought not to have been performed and includes those in which, for example, the wrong arm or leg has been operated on etc., but also cases in which it emerges retrospectively that, for example, a mastectomy has been performed on the basis of an incorrect diagnosis. The category "incorrect dressing or splinting" (4%) relates to situations in which, for example, a fracture is managed conservatively, hence without an operation being performed. This category also includes plaster casts, reduction and immobilisation of limbs.

The heading "injection, infusion and puncture techniques" (8%) may refer to situations involving diagnosis (e.g. incorrect injection of contrast media, lumbar puncture) or medication (incorrect application of an infusion in chemotherapy).

The same applies within the category "catheterisation and internal examination" (3%). Instances which come to mind here are those of cardiac catheterisation (diagnosis), laryngoscopy (diagnosis or operation), administering of enemas (medication), laparoscopy and arthroscopy (operation).
By "infection" (4.6%) is meant hospital viruses caught as a result of a lack of hygiene or sterility; this category also includes the hepatitis B infections in IVF treatment (54 instances).

In conclusion it is remarkable that in a good 10% of the cases investigated there is no question of any medico-technical basis. In many of these cases the injury claim is based on a defect in the equipment or the incorrect use thereof. It may also be the case with these claims that what is involved is a lack of consent or insufficient information. It also relates to injury claims

---

[13] In 19 cases of injury the medical context is not known. These cases have been excluded.

which involve other, general aspects of the treatment, e.g. inadequate nursing and/or care.
Then the question arises as to what extent the indemnity percentage differs depending on what has gone wrong in a medico-technical sense (Table 44)[14].

It emerges that a relatively large number of indemnities have been awarded in the case of intubation (60%; n = 111), operating material accidentally left *in situ* (73%; n = 45), infection (72%; n = 71), wrong blood or other fluids (58%; n = 12), wrong medication (54.5%; n = 22), procedure not indicated (49%; n = 69) and incorrect and/or late delivery (47% n = 17).

In percentage terms, few indemnities result from claims relating to the technique of catheterisation or internal examination (24%; n = 45), other aspects concerning medication, e.g. the side-effects of medicines or the wrong or unnecessary administration of medicines (20%; n = 15), together with other aspects relating to operations (19.5%; n = 87). This last named category refers to cases of injury involving an operative procedure, whereas it is not clear whether the injury is connected to the surgical technique.

In addition to the medical context the survey considered other aspects of the medical act/treatment. For example, we looked at how far attempts to obtain compensation were (also) based on a number of general aspects of the treatment. Here we consider an incorrect treatment protocol or method, inadequate nursing and/or care, or incorrect follow-up treatment or supervision. 319 of the cases investigated involve a so called general aspect (Table 45).
Here it should be pointed out that for each case a maximum of 1 general aspect has been ticked. If several aspects have been involved the most important has been chosen. In a good 20% of the 319 relevant cases it was a question of "incorrect treatment protocol or method". This includes situations in which, for example, a finger wound is sutured too quickly, causing infection or when, in a similar case, no hepatitis injection is given. One is also put in mind of cases in which the patient is not, or is incorrectly, referred or in which it was necessary to consult a different specialist. Finally, this category includes cases where a conservative therapy was wrongly applied.

In 18% of the abovementioned cases we are dealing with an incorrect follow-up treatment or supervision. These cases refer, for example, to operations which were, admittedly, properly performed, but which were followed post-

---

14 In addition to those 19 cases in which the medical context is not known, there is also 1 claim in respect of which it is not known whether an indemnity was paid or not. These cases have been omitted.

operatively by infection/fever/respiratory problems not noticed until later. These cases also include, for example, instances of where a limb has been dressed or put in a splint in the correct manner, but where, due to inadequate supervision, necrosis has arisen.

The percentage of indemnities for those claims in which a "general aspect" has played a role is relatively low, viz. an average of 26% (Table 46). Where "incorrect treatment protocol or method" is concerned, many claims are accepted, relatively speaking (40.6%; n = 69). We also observe that in the case of "inadequate result of treatment" relatively few claims are met (11.1%; n = 45).

After this it is interesting to examine the role played by improperly and/or wrongly used medical equipment (including medical aids) as a cause of medical injury or the bringing of an injury claim (Table 47).

It transpires that in 12% of the cases examined the claim was (also) based on defective equipment and/or the wrong use of same (n = 183). In 12% of cases we are dealing with a defect pure and simple in the medical equipment. A quarter of the cases involve incorrect use of the medical equipment. In the majority of the cases in question (61%) it is uncertain whether the origin of the claim is a defect in the equipment or the fact that it was wrongly used. About 2% of cases involve the fact that the equipment was not sterile. The percentage of awards in this category is a high one (67%) (Table 48). It appears that there is a high percentage of awards in the category "combination of defective and wrongly used equipment" (71%).

Attention is also drawn to the requirement for consent and the duty of information. To what extent are such aspects to be taken into account in the demand for compensation?

The survey reveals that in 96 of the cases investigated the claimant (also) cited a lack of consent or a failure in the duty of information (Table 49). Of those claims in which formal aspects play a part, the majority (72%) concern insufficient information about the medical procedure. Five cases involve a combination of lack of consent and insufficient information. In percentage terms the number of indemnities awarded in this category is low (average 27%) (Table 50).

Finally, this chapter on the medical aspects of claims devotes some attention to the nature of the injury sustained in connection with procedures performed in hospitals (Table 51)[15]. An investigation of these cases seldom reveals to what extent the injury is of a permanent nature, though this certainly *is* clear in the categories "amputation" and "death", and also in "pregnancy".

Moreover, it is difficult to draw a distinction between cases in which the injury should be considered as an injury purely and simply resulting from the medical procedure (iatrogenic injury) and those cases involving an injury which antedated the procedure, or an injury of a permanent kind, even though the treatment was correct. Moreover the injuries may differ somewhat in extent within a particular category. For example, the category known as "functional disorder or nervous lesions of the limbs" may include, for example, tingling in the fingers, but also paralysis of the arm(s) or leg(s).

In the interests of a methodical approach only one category of injury per claim investigated has been ticked. Table 51 (and 52) therefore provide some information on the most important injuries which have arisen after medical treatment.

Injury in the sense of a functional disorder or nervous lesions of the limbs is the largest category (26%), followed by the category "pain and/or discomfort" (15%). Even in this last category the variations are considerable: discomfort, for example, can be anything from a nasty bruise which soon goes to serious pains over a lengthy period. The table also shows that in 9% of claims there is some question of burns or other skin lesions. Even the category "death" occurs again (54 times) (3.6%).

In the case of claims accepted (Table 52)[16] a high percentage of indemnities are paid where brain damage is involved (86%; n = 7), functional disorders of other sense organs (75%; n = 4), inflammation and/or infection (51.5%; n = 103), dental lesions (60%; n = 148), burns or other skin lesions (62%; n = 133), fracture (52%; n = 27) and functional disorders of the stomach/intestine/oesophagus (52%; n = 44).
Relatively few indemnities have been paid in the case of functional disorders of sexual organs (21%; n = 19), functional disorders of the vocal chords (9%; N = 11), functional disorders of the ear (23%; n = 13) and death (17%; n = 54).

---

15 In 61 cases it is not known what injury occurred following medical treatment. These cases are left out of consideration here.

16 In addition to 61 cases in which the nature of the injury is not known, there is 1 claim in respect of which it is not known whether the claim was allowed. These cases have been disregarded here.

In addition to the foregoing considerations, the survey also addressed the question of whether an injury has led to one or more additional operations, which has been the case in 369 instances. This is almost 25% of the total number of cases investigated. Some of these cases involve a non-operative procedure wrongly performed which *has* had to be followed by surgical intervention. Usually, however, these are cases of incorrect acts during an operation, thus necessitating a fresh operation.

Chapter 5

CONCLUDING OBSERVATIONS

The number of medical injury claims for medical procedures in hospitals during the period 1980-1990 has increased sharply. The number of cases in which an indemnity has been paid has proportionally fallen and in absolute terms remains the same. The number of civil actions and proceedings before disciplinary tribunals initiated in the case of medical injury claims is at a low level and during the period covered by the survey even shows a downward curve. Most indemnities are below the *f* 5,000.-- mark and it is only in a few cases that very large ones are paid.

The increased number of injury claims cannot, incidentally, be viewed in isolation from a general social trend, viz. an increased maturity on the part of the citizen and consumer awareness. An additional factor of importance is the general popularisation of knowledge and science and, connected with this, the publicity generally accorded to this subject in the public health service.

The number of injury claims submitted in the Netherlands remains far behind that of the United States, a criterion also used for this comparison. In the United States the basis used is the number of injury claims per 100 doctors, while the number of injury claims per 100 occupied beds is used as a unit of calculation. The major insurer The St. Paul and Marine Insurance Company reports that in 1985 17.9 claims per 100 doctors were submitted[1].

Transposed to the situation in the Netherlands this would lead to a greater number of claims per year than those which were made during the 10 year period covered by the survey. It must be remembered that this survey relates only to injury claims made in respect of medical acts in hospitals. But, as is well known, *most* medical injuries occur in hospitals. However, even when the percentage just mentioned is applied only to medical specialists (5700 in 1985; and even in the years since then this number has remained pretty much the same) it would, transposed to the Netherlands, mean more than 1,000 injury claims a year. Even if we apply as a yardstick the number of

---

1 *Vide* Stolker C.J.J.M., From Doctor to Lawyer - Liability for Medical Errors in America, Utrecht, 1989, p. 11.

medical injury claims per 100 occupied beds - in the U.S. figures are cited which vary between 3.4 and 8.2 claims per 100 occupied beds[2] - it would, as far as the Netherlands are concerned, also lead to a number of injury claims each year many times in excess of the number of claims made during the years covered by the survey. The number of claims submitted also appears relatively low when related to the total number of procedures performed in Dutch hospitals. This is also true if the figure is related to the number of admissions and the number of full-time equivalents of medical specialists.

The average indemnity paid out per injury claim admits of no comparison at all. Our data reveal that in the Netherlands during the period covered by the survey the average indemnity for surgeons is *f* 19,861.-- and for non-surgical specialists *f* 28,010.--. The general average is *f* 19,825.--. The median in these categories is considerably lower (*f* 6,366.-- and *f* 2,500.-- respectively). The modus is *f* 10,000.-- and *f* 5,000.-- respectively. In the United States the average indemnity is much higher, but the number of very high indemnities is appreciably larger.

More important, however, is the fact that in the United States the number of claims in which an indemnity has been paid has risen by no less than 264% during the period from 1980 to 1987. Manual recently produced figures which point in the same direction and which also showed, incidentally, that in the United States a much larger number of claims reach the courts[3].

Our survey of cases reveals that such tendencies were not present in the Netherlands during the period covered by the work. This does not mean, incidentally, that there is no resemblance to the United States. The average time taken to settle a medical injury claim bears a striking similarity to the Netherlands, where the average time emerges as approximately 20 months.

There is, by the way, hardly any difference in the time taken to settle claims, whether an indemnity is paid or not. In the United States insurers take about a month longer on average and the average duration of settlement is 21 months. This lengthy period raises the question of whether injury claims could be dealt with more simply and hence more quickly. With this in mind, reference was made earlier by the Dutch National Council of Public Health, among other bodies, to the possibility of setting up a disputes board for this purpose. On the bases of the material gathered from the survey we shall

---

2 Op cit. p. 12

3 B. Manual What may happen if there is no change in the U.K. system? In: Compensation and Accountability, London 1992, pp. 89-109.

address this question in greater detail in a separate paper[4].
The qualification just made does not mean that we in the Netherlands can calmly allow developments to take their course. To adopt such an attitude may perhaps lead to the number of claims rising further and also, possibly, to a rise in the number of accepted claims. The injury claims now being made should teach us a thing or two on the subject of prevention and quality care in hospitals.

An analysis of the medico-technical basis of injury claims shows that a significant number of these originate in procedural errors. This may be illustrated with the aid of the following three examples. To begin with, nearly 3% of the injury claims are related to a failure to remove operating material accidentally left *in situ*. In 73% of this category of injury claims, according to the survey, an indemnity is paid. These, however, are avoidable errors.

Secondly, we have injury claims resulting from defective equipment or from the incorrect use of medical equipment or aids. These causes seem to be at issue in approximately 12% of all claims. In most of them, incidentally, what is involved is a combination of defects and incorrect use. The survey reveals that in nearly 67% of cases these claims have led to an indemnity being paid. Finally, it emerges that in approximately 6% of cases the patient was inadequately informed or consent was not obtained. The number of cases in which these failures led to an indemnity being paid is smaller than either of the two categories just mentioned, yet still amounts to 27%. These, too, belong to the avoidable causes of injury claims. This last one also applies to a number of other categories of injury claims.

Finally, it may be remarked that a proper settlement of medical injury claims will also look to see what lessons can be drawn from them. This is in the interests of all parties involved - doctors, patients and insurers. For this reason it is of great importance to link the settlement of medical injury claims to quality care in hospitals.

The figures presented make it difficult to forecast for the near future. A significant role should be attached to the fact that we are dealing here with a so called dark number of errors and accidents in the public health service, to which a number of recent domestic and foreign publications point[5,6]. This,

---

[4] National Council of Public Health, Recommendation on the meeting of Claims in the Public Health Service, Zoetermeer 1989.

[5] Medical Care and Medical Injury in the State of New York; a pilot study, Cambridge, Massachusetts, April 1987.

too, is an important reason why matters should not calmly be allowed to run their course, but rather that attention should continue to be paid to quality care in Dutch hospitals.

[6] Tempelaar A.F., Safety and Risk in the Public Health Service; Epidemiological Aspects of Iatrogenic Injury, Groningen 1991.

References

Aller, H.B. van (red.), *Schadevergoeding na medische fout, geluk bij een ongeluk?*, Faculteit der Rechtsgeleerdheid, Universiteit van Amsterdam 1988.

Asser, W.D.H., *Stelplicht, bewijslastverdeling en medische aansprakelijkheid in het Nederlandse recht*, Tijdschrift voor Gezondheidsrecht 1991, p. 62-76.

Beer, J.M., S.C.J.J. Kortmann, L.H.D.J. Booy, *Aansprakelijkheid voor medische fouten vanuit juridisch oogpunt bezien*, Koninklijke Vermande, Lelystad 1991.

Boon, L., *Fouten in de Gezondheidszorg*, Stichting Sympoz, Amsterdam 1988.

Brennan, T.A. et.al., *Incidence of advense events and negligence in hospitalized patients*, N.Engl. J. med. 1991, 324:370-6.

Hubben, J.H., L.G. Angenent, *De afwikkeling van medische schadeclaims*, in: J.H. Hubben (red.), Rechtsbijstand in de gezondheidszorg, De Tijdstroom, Lochem 1989.

Hubben, J.H., *De civiele rechter en medische schadeclaims*. In: Grenzen aan zorg; zorgen aan de grens, Alphen a/d Rijn 1990.

Kiezen en delen, rapport van de Commissie Keuzen in de zorg (commissie Dunning), 's-Gravenhage, mei 1991.

Knol, R.C., *Vergoeding van letselschade volgens huidig en komend recht*, Tjeenk Willink, Zwolle 1986.

Manual, B., *What may happen if there is no change in the US-system?* in: Compensation and Accountabilty, London 1992.

Medical Care and Medical Injury in the State of New York: a pilot study, Cambridge, Massachusets, april 1987.

Medische aansprakelijkheid onbetaalbaar perspectief. Uitgave VVAA ter gelegenheid van een symposium gehouden op 14 februari 1992 te Ede.

Mol, B.A.J.M. de, *Medisch letsel in het ziekenhuis*, een verkennende studie, Kluwer, Deventer 1988.

Nationale Raad voor de Volksgezondheid, *Rapport verkennende studie patiëntenletselverzekering*, Zoetermeer 1989.

Nationale Raad voor de Volksgezondheid, *Standaard-classificatie medisch specialistische verrichtingen*, Zoetermeer 1990 (2e druk).

Nationale Raad voor de Volksgezondheid, *Advies klachtenopvang in de gezondheidszorg*, Zoetermeer 1989.

Sluyters, B., *De aansprakelijkheid van arts en ziekenhuis*, Deventer 1984.
Stolker, C.J.J.M., *Aansprakelijkheid van de arts, in het bijzonder voor mislukte sterilisatie*, Deventer 1988.
Stolker, C.J.J.M., *Van arts naar advocaat, aansprakelijkheid voor medische fouten in Amerika*, Utrecht/Deventer 1989.

Tempelaar, A.F., *Veiligheid en risico in de gezondheidszorg, Epidemiologische aspecten van iatrogene schade*, Groningen 1991.

List of figures

List of tables

Appendix 1

Tables

Table 1 Injury claims by year reported

	number	%	valid%	cum %
1980	9	0,6	0,6	0,6
1981	20	1,3	1,3	1,9
1982	48	3,1	3,1	5,0
1983	103	6,6	6,6	11,6
1984	152	9,8	9,8	21,4
1985	175	11,3	11,3	32,7
1986	201	13,0	13,0	45,7
1987	190	12,3	12,3	57,9
1988	313	20,2	20,2	78,1
1989	339	21,9	21,9	100,0
Total	1550	100,0	100,0	

Valid cases: 1550

Year reported: year in which injury claim submitted

Table 2 Injury claims by year of injury and year reported

Year of	year reported										
injury	1980	1981	1982	1983	1984	1985	1986	1987	1988	1989	row total
1980	9	12	9	5	2	2	1	2	3	1	46
	19,6	26,1	19,6	10,9	4,3	4,3	2,2	4,3	6,5	2,2	3,0
	100,0	63,2	19,1	4,9	1,3	1,1	0,5	1,1	1,0	0,3	
	0,6	0,8	0,6	0,3	0,1	0,1	0,1	0,1	0,2	0,1	
1981		7	17	13	5	4	8	4	2	3	63
		11,1	27,0	20,6	7,9	6,3	12,7	6,3	3,2	4,8	4,1
		36,8	36,2	12,7	3,3	2,3	4,0	2,1	0,6	0,9	
		0,5	1,1	0,8	0,3	0,3	0,5	0,3	0,1	0,2	
1982			21	40	19	10	9	1	3	3	106
			19,8	37,7	17,9	9,4	8,5	0,9	2,8	2,8	6,9
			44,7	39,2	12,6	5,7	4,5	0,5	1,0	0,9	
			1,4	2,6	1,2	0,7	0,6	0,1	0,2	0,2	
1983				44	68	21	7	2	8	6	156
				28,2	43,6	13,5	4,5	1,3	5,1	3,8	10,1
				43,1	45,0	12,1	3,5	1,1	2,6	1,8	
				2,9	4,4	1,4	0,5	0,1	0,5	0,4	
1984					57	61	23	10	5	6	162
					35,2	37,7	14,2	6,2	3,1	3,7	10,5
					37,7	35,1	11,5	5,3	1,6	1,8	
					3,7	4,0	1,5	0,7	0,3	0,4	
1985						76	71	24	12	11	194
						39,2	36,6	12,4	6,2	5,7	12,6
						43,7	35,5	12,8	3,9	3,3	
						4,9	4,6	1,6	0,8	0,7	
1986							81	67	34	18	200
							40,5	33,5	17,0	9,0	13,0
							40,5	35,6	10,9	5,3	
							5,3	4,4	2,2	1,2	
1987								78	109	40	227
								34,4	48,0	17,6	14,8
								41,5	35,0	11,9	
								5,1	7,1	2,6	
1988 abs. number									135	118	253
row %									53,4	46,6	16,4
column %									43,4	35,0	
total %									8,8	7,7	
1989										131	131
										100,0	8,5
										38,9	
											8,5
column	9	19	47	102	151	174	200	188	311	337	1538
total	0,6	1,2	3,1	6,6	9,8	11,3	13,0	12,2	20,2	21,9	100,0

Valid cases: 1538; Missing cases: 12. Year reported: year in which injury claim submitted. Year of injury: year in which injury occurred

Table 3 Injury claims by year reported and whether or not indemnity paid

absolute number row % column % total % year reported	indemnity yes	 no	 row- total
1980	5	4	9
	55,6	44,4	0,6
	0,8	0,4	
	0,3	0,3	
1981	12	8	20
	60,0	40,0	1,3
	1,9	0,9	
	0,8	0,5	
1982	21	27	48
	43,8	56,3	3,1
	3,4	2,9	
	1,4	1,7	
1983	44	58	102
	43,1	56,9	6,6
	7,0	6,3	
	2,8	3,7	
1984	80	72	152
	52,6	47,4	9,8
	12,8	7,8	
	5,2	4,6	
1985	82	93	175
	46,9	53,1	11,3
	13,1	10,1	
	5,3	6,0	
1986	75	126	201
	37,3	62,7	13,0
	12,0	13,7	
	4,8	8,1	
1987	84	106	190
	44,2	55,8	12,3
	13,4	11,5	
	5,4	6,8	
1988	141	172	313
	45,0	55,0	20,2
	22,5	18,6	
	9,1	11,1	
1989	82	257	339
	24,2	75,8	21,9
	13,1	27,8	
	5,3	16,6	
column	626	923	1549
total	40,4	59,6	100,0

Valid cases: 1549 Missing cases: 1

Table 4 Way in which case closed when claim rejected

	number	%	valid %
no action following rejection of claim by insurer	299	19,3	54,2
no action following rejection of claim by neutral expert phycisian	40	2,6	7,2
no action following dismissal of civil law claim	4	0,3	0,7
no action following dismissal of complaint by medical disciplinary tibunal	16	1,0	2,9
no further action following dismissal of complaint by medical disciplinary tribunal	3	0,2	0,5
no further action following upholding of complaint by medical disciplinary tribunal	4	0,3	0,7
no further action following admission by insurer	10	0,6	1,8
no further action after claim reported	90	5,8	16,3
claim withdrawn	33	2,1	6,0
injury not covered by policy	9	0,6	1,6
more than one insurer	7	0,5	1,3
other	37	2,4	6,7
n/a	998	64,4	missing
Total	1550	100,0	100,0

Valid cases 552 Missing cases 998

Table 5 Level of indemity in categories

f	number	%	valid %	cum %
< = 1000	119	7,7	19,0	19,0
1001-2000	77	5,0	12,3	31,3
2001-3000	57	3,7	9,1	40,4
3001-4000	38	2,5	6,1	46,5
4001-5000	42	2,7	6,7	53,2
5001-10000	97	6,3	15,5	68,7
10001-20000	74	4,8	11,8	80,5
20001-50000	55	3,5	8,8	89,3
50001-100000	49	3,2	7,8	97,1
100001-200000	11	0,7	1,8	98,9
200001-999998	7	0,5	1,1	100,0
n/a	924	59,6	missing	
total	1550	100,0	100,0	

Valid cases: 626 Missing cases: 924

Table 6 Injury cases in which *f* 100,000.-- or more is paid out

year closed	indemnity	property damage costs	compensation for pain and suffering	compensation for pain and suffering in NLG
1981	225.000	66,67	33,33	± 75.000,--
1984	109.500	31,51	68,49	75.000,--
1987	104.300	71,24	28,76	30.000,--
1987	110.000	45,45	54,55	60.000,--
1988	115.525	84,85	15,15	± 17.500,--
1989	119.674	93,52	6,48	7.750,--
1989	160.000	84,38	15,63	25.000,--
1989	260.000	75,00	25,00	65.000,--
1989	640.000	88,28	11,72	75.000,--
1989	111.500	46,19	53,81	60.000,--
1989	115.000	-	-	-
1990	100.000	-	-	-
1990	100.274	50,14	49,86	50.000,--
1990	154.713	61,22	38,78	60.000,--
1990	752.500	-	-	-
open	100.000	-	-	-
open	129.270	53,59	46,41	60.000,--
open	315.000	76,19	23,81	75.000,--
open	399.859	81,24	18,76	75.000,--
open	625.000	84,00	16,00	100.000,--

- = not known

Valid cases: 20

Table 7 Level of indemnity in NLG by year reported

abs.number row-tot. Kol. % Tot. % **Year of report**	**level of indemnity in NLG** <=1000	1001- 2000	2001- 3000	3001- 4000	4001- 5000	5001- 10000	10001- 20000	20001- 50000	50001 100000	100001 200000	200001 9999998	row total
1980						2	1		2			5
						40,0	20,0		40,0			0,8
						2,1	1,4	4,1				
						0,3	0,2		0,3			
1981		2				2	1	1	3	1	2	12
		16,7				16,7	8.3	8,3	25,0	8,3	16,7	1,9
		2,6				2,1	1,4	1,8	6,1	9,1	28,6	
		0,3				0,3	0,2	0,2	0,5	0,2	0,3	
1982	5	3	2	2	1	2	1		5			21
	23,8	14,3	9,5	9,5	4,8	9,5	4,8		23,8			3,4
	4,2	3,9	3,5	5,3	2,4	2,1	1,4		10,2			
	0,8	0,5	0,3	0,3	0,2	0,3	0,2		0,8			
1983	8	5	3	2	2	5	9	4	4	1	1	44
	18,2	11,4	6,8	4,5	4,5	11,4	20,5	9,1	9,1	2,3	2,3	7,0
	6,7	6,5	5,3	5.3	4,8	5,2	12,2	7,3	8,2	9,1	14,3	
	1.3	0,8	0,5	0,3	0,3	0,8	1,4	0,6	0,6	0,2	0,2	
1984	12	6	6	5	3	8	10	9	13	7	1	80
	15,0	7,5	7,5	6,3	3,8	10,0	12,5	11,3	16,3	8,8	1,3	12,8
	10,1	7,8	10,5	13,2	7,1	8,2	13,5	16.4	26,5	63,6	14,3	
	1,9	1,0	1,0	0.8	0,5	1,3	1,6	1,4	2,1	1,1	0,2	
1985	12	11	10	3	6	11	15	8	6			82
	14,6	13,4	12,2	2,7	7,3	13,4	18,3	9,8	7,3			13,1
	10,1	14,3	17,5	7,9	14,3	11,3	20,3	14,5	12,2			
	1,9	1,8	1,6	0,5	1.0	1,8	2,4	1,3	1,0			
1986	16	9	10	3	4	11	5	11	3	1	2	75
	21,3	12,0	13,3	4,0	5,3	14.7	6,7	14,7	4,0	1,3	2,7	12,0
	13,4	11,7	17,5	7,9	9,5	11,3	6,8	20,0	6,1	9,1	28,6	
	2,6	1.4	1,6	0,5	0,6	1,8	0,8	1,8	0,5	0,2	0,3	
1987	15	14	4	5	9	13	10	7	5	1	1	84
	17.9	16,7	4,8	6,0	10,7	15,5	11,9	8,3	6,0	1,2	1,2	13,4
	12.6	18,2	7,0	13,2	21,4	13,4	13,5	12,7	10,2	9,1	14,3	
	2,4	2.2	0,6	0,8	1,4	2,1	1,6	1,1	0,8	0,2	0,2	
1988	28	18	9	14	14	22	18	13	5			141
	19,9	12,8	6,4	9,9	9,9	15,6	12,8	9,2	3,5			22,5
	23,5	23,4	15,8	36,8	33,3	22,7	24,3	23,6	10,2			
	4.5	2,9	1,4	2,2	2,2	3,5	2,9	2,1	0,8			
1989	23	9	13	4	3	21	4	2	3			82
	28,0	11,0	15,9	4,9	3,7	25,6	4,9	2,4	3,7			13,1
	19,3	11,7	22,8	10,5	7,1	21,6	5,4	3,6	6,1			
	3,7	1,4	2,1	0,6	0,5	3,4	0,6	0,3	0,5			
Column	119	77	57	38	42	97	74	55	49	11	7	626
Total	19,0	12,3	9,1	6,1	6,7	15,5	11.8	8,8	7,8	1,8	1,1	100,0

Valid cases: 626 Missing cases: 924

Table 8 Injury claims by level of pain and suffering payments

	number	%	valid %	cum %
not known	187	12,1	39,8	39,8
< = 1000	34	2,2	7,2	47,0
1001-2000	24	1,5	5,1	52,1
2001-3000	39	2,5	8,3	60,4
3001-4000	23	1,5	4,9	65,3
4001-5000	26	1,7	5,5	70,9
5001-10000	50	3,2	10,6	81,5
10001-20000	34	2,2	7,2	88,7
20001-50000	37	2,4	7,9	96,6
50001-100000	16	1,0	3,4	100,0
n/a		1080	69,7	missing
Total		1550	100,0	100,0

Valid cases: 470 Missing cases: 1080

Table 9 Relationship between reserve and indemnity; the reserve is expressed as a percentage of the indemnity

% of the indemnity	number	%	valid %
0-75	47	8,6	10
75-125	12	22,3	26
125-200	91	16,6	19,5
200-500	127	23,2	27,3
500-1000	46	8,4	9,8
1000-2500	26	4,7	5,5
2500-± 5000	7	1,3	1,5
n/a	80	14,8	missing
Total	546	100,0	100,0

Valid cases: 546 Missing cases: 80

Table 10 Injury claims from the standpoint of liability

	number	%	valid %
admitted	497	32,1	42,4
rejected	675	43,5	57,6
not known	378	24,4	missing
Total	1550	100,0	100,0

Valid cases: 1172 Missing cases: 378

Table 11 Injury claims by year reported and whether or not involving civil proceedings

absolute / row % / column % / total %	civil proceedings: yes	no	row total
Year of report			
1980	2	7	9
	22,2	77,8	0,6
	3,2	0,5	
	0,1	0,5	
1981	3	17	20
	15,0	85,0	1,3
	4,8	1,1	
	0,2	1,1	
1982	4	44	48
	8,3	91,7	3,1
	6,3	3,0	
	0,3	2,8	
1983	6	96	102
	5,9	94,1	6,6
	9,5	6,5	
	0,4	6,2	
1984	6	146	152
	3,9	96,1	9,8
	9,5	9,8	
	0,4	9,4	
1985	7	168	175
	4,0	96,0	11,3
	11,1	11,3	
	0,5	10,9	
1986	11	190	201
	5,5	94,5	13,0
	17,5	12,8	
	0,7	12,3	
1987	9	181	190
	4,7	95,3	12,3
	14,3	12,2	
	0,6	11,7	
1988	10	303	313
	3,2	96,8	20,2
	15,9	20,4	
	0,6	19,6	
1989	5	333	338
	1,5	98,5	21,8
	7,9	22,4	
	0,3	21,5	
Column	63	1485	1548
Total	4,1	95,9	100,0

Valid cases: 1548 Missing cases: 2

Table 12 Injury claims by year reported and whether or not involving disciplinary tribunal proceedings

absolute row % column % total %	tribunal proceedings yes	 no	 row total
Year of report			
1980	1	8	9
	11,1	88,9	0,6
	1,1	0,6	
	0,1	0,5	
1981	2	18	20
	10,0	90,0	1,3
	2,2	1,2	
	0,1	1,2	
1982	2	46	48
	4,2	95,8	3,1
	2,2	3,2	
	0,1	3,0	
1983	5	96	101
	5,0	95,0	6,5
	5,4	6,6	
	0,3	6,2	
1984	12	140	152
	7,9	92,1	9,8
	13,0	9,6	
	0,8	9,1	

Valid cases: 1545 Missing cases: 5

absolute row % column % total %	tribunal proceedings yes	 no	 row total
Year of report			
1985	8	167	175
	4,6	95,4	11,3
	8,7	11,5	
	0,5	10,8	
1986	18	182	200
	9,0	91,0	12,9
	19,6	12,5	
	1.2	11,8	
1987	12	178	190
	6,3	93,7	12,3
	13,0	12,3	
	0,8	11,5	
1988	12	301	313
	3,8	96,2	20,3
	13,0	20,7	
	0,8	19,5	
1989	20	317	337
	5,9	94,1	21,8
	21,7	21,8	
	1,3	20,5	
Column	92	1453	1545
Total	6,0	94,0	100,0

Table 13 Injury claims by outcome of disciplinary tribunal proceedings

	number	%	valid %
Not known	23	1,8	25,0
upheld	23	1,5	25,0
dismissed	43	2,8	46,7
withdrawn	3	0,2	3,2
n/a	1458	93,7	missing
Total	1550	100,0	100,0

Valid cases: 92 Missing cases: 1458

Table 14 Injury claims by disciplinary tribunal proceedings and wheter or not indemnity paid

absolute row % column % total %	indemnity yes	 no	 row total
Disciplinary tribunal proceedings			
yes	19 20,7 3,0 1,2	73 79,3 7,9 4,7	92 6,0
no	607 41,8 97,0 39,3	846 58,2 92,1 54,8	1453 94,0
Column Total	626 40,5	919 59,5	1545 100,0

Valid cases: 1545 Missing cases: 5

Table 15 Injury claims by year reported and whether or not involving complaint to medical inspectorate

absolute / row % / column % / total %	complaint to inspectorate: yes	no	row total
Year reported			
1980	1	8	9
	11,1	88,9	0,6
	2,2	0,5	
	0,1	0,5	
1981		20	20
		100,0	1,3
		1,3	
		1,3	
1982	1	47	48
	2,1	97,9	3,1
	2,2	3,1	
	0,1	3,0	
1983	4	98	102
	3,9	96,1	6,6
	8,7	6,5	
	0,3	6,3	
1984	10	142	152
	6,6	93,4	9,8
	21,7	9,5	
	0,6	9,2	
1985	3	172	175
	1,7	98,3	11,3
	6,5	11,5	
	0,2	11,1	
1986	5	195	200
	2,5	97,5	12,9
	10,9	13,0	
	0,3	12,6	
1987	4	186	190
	2,1	97,9	12,3
	8,7	12,4	
	0,3	12,0	
1988	6	306	312
	1,9	98,1	20,2
	13,0	20,4	
	0,4	19,8	
1989	12	327	339
	3,5	96,5	21,9
	26,1	21,8	
	0,8	21,1	
Column	46	1501	1547
Total	3,0	97,0	100,0

Valid cases: 1547 Missing cases: 3

Table 16 Injury claims by complaint to medical inspectorate and whether or not indemnity paid

absolute row % column % total %	indemnity yes	 no	 row total
complaint to inspectorate			
yes	11 23,9 1,8 0,7	35 76,1 3,8 2,3	46 3,0
no	615 41,0 98,2 39,8	886 59,0 96,2 57,3	1501 97,0
Column Total	626 40,5	921 59,5	1547 100,0

Valid cases: 1547 Missing cases: 3

Table 17 Injury claims by whether or not civil proceedings involved and whether or not involving disciplinary tribunal proceedings

absolute row % column % total %	indemnity yes	 no	 row total
civil proceedings			
yes	10 15,9 10,9 0,6	53 84,1 3,7 3,4	63 4,1
no	82 5,5 89,1 5,3	1399 94,5 96,3 90,6	1481 95,9
Column Total	92 6,0	1452 94,0	1544 100,0

Valid cases: 1544 Missing cases: 6

Table 18 Injury claims by legal assistance

	number	%	valid %
	680	43,9	44,1
claims settlement agency	24	1,5	1,6
legal defence insurance	43	2,8	2,8
trade union legal defence	63	4,1	4,1
other	113	7,3	7,3
no assistance	619	39,9	40,1
not known	8	0,5	missing
Total	1550	100,0	100,0

Valid cases: 1542 Missing cases: 8

Table 19 Injury claims by year reported and whether or not with legal assistance

absolute row % column % total %	legal assistance yes	no	row total
Year reported			
1980	7	2	9
	77,8	22,2	0,6
	0,8	0,3	
	0,5	0,1	
1981	18	2	20
	90,0	10,0	1,3
	2,0	0,3	
	1,2	0,1	
1982	23	25	48
	47,9	52,1	3,1
	2,5	4,0	
	1,5	1,6	
1983	66	35	101
	65,3	34,7	6,5
	7,2	5,7	
	4,3	2,3	
1984	84	68	152
	55,3	44,7	9,9
	9,1	11,0	
	5,4	4,4	
1985	93	81	174
	53,4	46,6	11,3
	10,1	13,1	
	6,0	5,3	
1986	113	87	200
	56,5	43,5	13,0
	12,2	14,1	
	7,3	5,6	
1987	113	76	189
	59,8	40,2	12,3
	12,2	12,3	
	7,3	4,9	
1988	194	117	311
	62,4	37,6	20,2
	21,0	18,9	
	12,6	7,6	
1989	212	126	338
	62,7	37,3	21,9
	23,0	20,4	
	13,7	8,2	
Column Total	923	619	1542
	59,9	40,1	100,0

Valid cases: 1542 Missing cases: 8

Table 20 Injury claims by legal assistance and whether or not indemnity paid

absolute row % column % total %	indemnity yes	no	row total
lawyer	286 42,1 45,8 18,5	394 57,9 43,0 25,6	680 44,1
claims settlement agency	10 41,7 1,6 0,6	14 58,3 1,5 0,9	24 1,6
legal defence insurance	18 41,9 2,9 1,2	25 58,1 2,7 1,6	43 2,8
trade union legal defence	23 36,5 3,7 1,5	40 63,5 4,4 2,6	63 4,1
other	44 38,9 7,0 2,9	69 61,1 7,5 4,5	113 7,3
no assistance	244 39,4 39,0 15,8	375 60,6 40,9 24,3	619 40,1
Column Total	625 40,5	917 59,5	1542 100,0

Valid cases: 1542 Missing cases: 8

Table 21 Injury claims following enlistment of neutral expert physician

	number	%	valid %
insurer	40	2,6	10,3
claimant	16	1,0	4,1
joint(ly)	314	20,3	80,9
CAMA*	3	0,2	0,8
claims agent's office	1	0,1	0,3
judicial authority	11	0,7	2,8
inspectorate	3	0,2	0,8
n/a	1162	75,0	missing
Total	1550	100,0	100,0

Valid cases: 388 Missing cases: 1162

* Advising Commission Medical Liability

Table 22 Injury claims by terms of reference of neutral expert physician

	number	%	valid %
legal liability judgment/causal connection	240	15,5	67,0
permanent incapacity judgment/ final condition	62	4,0	17,3
judgment on both	52	3,4	14,5
other	4	0,3	1,1
n/a	1192	76,9	missing
Total	1550	100,0	100,0

Valid cases: 358 Missing cases: 1192

Table 23 Injury claims following enlistment of second neutral expert physician

	number	%	valid %
insurer	3	0,2	6,1
claimant	1	0,1	2,0
joint(ly)	35	2,3	71,4
CAMA*	1	0,1	2,0
judicial authority	9	0,6	18,4
n/a	1501	96,8	missing
Total	1550	100,0	100,0

Valid cases: 49 Missing cases: 1501

* Advising Commission Medical Liability

Table 24 Injury claims by person submitting claim

	number	%	valid %
patient	1201	77,5	80,5
family	62	4,0	4,2
parents	164	10,6	11,0
other	21	1,4	1,4
no claimant	44	2,8	2,9
not known	58	3,7	missing
Total	1550	100,0	100,0

Valid cases: 1492 Missing cases: 58

Table 25 Injury claims by third parties according to person making claim

	number	%	valid %
not known	6	0,4	6,7
sickness costs insurance	52	3,4	57,8
trade association	9	0,6	10,0
employer	8	0,5	8,9
other	15	1,0	16,7
n/a	1460	94,2	missing
Total	1550	100,0	100,0

Valid cases: 90 Missing cases: 1460

Table 26 Injury claims by third parties by level of indemnity

f	number	%	valid %	cum %
<=1000	2	2,2	4,2	4,2
1001-2000	9	10,0	18,8	22,9
2001-3000	3	3,3	6,3	29,2
3001-4000	2	2,2	4,2	33,3
4001-5000	3	3,3	6,3	39,6
5001-10000	12	13,3	25,0	64,6
10001-20000	6	6,7	12,5	77,1
20001-50000	7	7,8	14,6	91,7
50001-100000	3	3,3	6,3	97,9
100001-200000	1	1,1	2,1	100,0
n/a	42	46,7	missing	
Total	90	100,0	100,0	

Valid cases: 48 Missing cases: 42

Table 27 Injury claims by sex

	number	%	valid %
male	615	39,7	39,9
female	928	59,9	60,1
not known	7	0,5	missing
Total	1550	100,0	100,0

Valid cases: 1543 Missing cases: 7

Table 28 Injury claims by age

	number	%	valid %
0-10 year(s)	103	6,6	7,3
11-20 year(s)	107	6,9	7,6
21-30 year(s)	189	12,2	13,3
31-40 year(s)	331	21,4	23,4
41-50 year(s)	254	16,4	17,9
51-60 year(s)	208	13,4	14,7
61-70 year(s)	145	9,4	10,2
>= 71 year(s)	80	5,2	5,6
not known	133	8,6	missing
Total	1550	100,0	100,0

Valid cases: 1417 Missing cases: 133

Table 29 Injury claims by sex and whether or not indemnity paid

absolute row % column % total %	indemnity yes	 no	 row total
male	198 32,2 31,8 12,8	416 67,8 45,3 27,0	614 39,8
female	425 45,8 68,2 27,6	503 54,2 54,7 32,6	928 60,2
Column Total	623 40,4	919 59,6	1542 100,0

Valid cases: 1542 Missing cases: 8

Table 30 Injury claims by profession/occupation

	number	%	valid %
wage earner	268	17,3	64,1
self-employed	48	3,1	11,5
unemployed	2	0,1	0,5
incapacitated for work	20	1,3	4,8
student	27	1,7	6,5
housewife	51	3,3	12,2
other	2	0,1	0,5
n/a	1132	73,0	missing
Total	1550	100,0	100,0

Valid cases: 418 Missing cases: 1132

Table 31 Injury claims by type of hospital

	number	%	valid %	cum %
teaching hospital	343	22,1	22,2	22,2
general hospital	1164	75,1	75,3	97,5
cancer hospital	16	1,0	1,0	98,5
children's hospital	4	0,3	0,3	98,8
eye hospital	5	0,3	0,3	99,1
other	14	0,9	0,9	100,0
not known	4	0,3	missing	
Total	1550	100,0	100,0	100,0

Valid cases: 1546 Missing cases: 4

Table 32 Injury claims by type of hospital and whether or not indemnity paid

absolute row % column % total %	indemnity yes	 no	 row total
type of hospital			
	153	189	342
university hospital	44,7	55,3	22,1
		24,5	20,5
		9,9	12,2
	456	708	1164
general	39,2	60,8	75,3
		73,0	77,0
		29,5	45,8
	6	10	16
cancer hospital	37,5	62,5	1,0
		1,0	1,1
		0,4	0,6
	2	2	4
children's hospital	50,0	50,0	0,3
		0,3	0,2
		0,1	0,1
	5		5
eye hospital	100,0		0,3
		0,8	
		0,3	
	3	11	14
other	21,4	78,6	0,9
		0,5	1,2
		0,2	0,7
Column	625	920	1545
Total	40,5	59,5	100,0

Valid cases: 1545 Missing cases: 5

Table 33 Injury claims by classification of medical procedure

	number	%
diagnostic	296	19,1
medication	67	4,3
operative	680	43,9
confinement	47	3,0
other therapeutic procedure	406	26,2
other	54	3,5
Total	1550	100,0

Valid cases: 1550 Missing cases: 0

Table 34 Injury claims by classification of medical procedure and whether or not indemnity paid

absolute row % column % total %	indemnity yes	 no	 row total
medical procedure			
	103	193	296
diagnostic	34,8	65,2	19,1
	16,5	20,9	
	6,6	12,5	
	34	33	67
medication	50,7	49,3	4,3
	5,4	3,6	
	2,2	2,1	
	255	424	679
operative	37,6	62,4	43,8
	40,7	45,9	
	16,5	27,4	
	23	24	47
confinement	48,9	51,1	3,0
	3,7	2,6	
	1,5	1,5	
	195	211	406
other therapeutic	48,0	52,0	26,2
procedure	31,2	22,9	
	12,6	13,6	
	16	38	54
other	29,6	0,4	3,5
	2,6	4,1	
	1,0	2,5	
Column	626	923	1549
Total	40,4	59,6	100,0

Valid cases: 1549 Missing cases: 1

Table 35 Injury claims by type of operation

	Number	%	valid %
not known	21	1,4	3,1
nervous system	30	1,9	4,4
endocrine glands	10	0,6	1,5
eyes	11	0,7	1,6
ears	23	1,5	3,4
nasal cavity & paranasal sinus	9	0,6	1,3
oral cavity	38	2,5	5,6
throat	18	1,2	2,6
lungs and bronchial tubes	2	0,1	0,3
heart	15	1,0	2,2
blood vessels	30	1,9	4,4
blood and lymphatic system	13	0,8	1,9
digestive tract	70	4,5	10,3
urinary tract	28	1,8	4,1
male sexual organs	23	1,5	3,4
female sexual organs	101	6,5	14,9
musculo-skeletal system	196	12,6	28,8
breasts	18	1,2	2,6
skin and subcutis	24	1,5	3,5
no operation	870	56,1	missing
Total	1550	100,0	100,0

Valid cases: 680 Missing cases: 870

Table 36 Injury claims by other therapeutic procedures

	number	%	valid %
not known	24	1,5	5,6
anaesthetic	162	10,5	38,0
dressings/splints etc.	60	3,9	14,1
treatment of wounds	12	0,8	2,8
other	114	7,4	26,8
IVF	54	3,5	18,7
n/a	1144	72,5	missing
Total	1550	100,0	100,0

Valid cases: 406 Missing cases: 1144

Table 37 Injury claims by operator and whether or not indemnity paid

absolute row % column % total %	**indemnity** yes	no	row total
operator			
	347	579	926
surgical	37,5	62,5	61,9
	57,5	64,8	
	23,2	38,7	2,00
	138	222	360
non-surgical	38,3	61,7	24,0
		22,8	24,9
		9,2	14,8
	19	23	42
non-specialist doctor	45,2	54,8	2,8
	3,1	2,6	
	1,3	1,5	
	97	61	158
other	61,4	38,6	10,6
	16,1	6,8	
	6,5	4,1	
	3	8	11
no operator	27,3	72,7	0,7
	0,5	0,9	
	0,2	0,5	
Column	604	893	1497
Total	40,3	59,7	100,0

Valid cases: 1497 Missing cases: 53

Table 38 Injury claims relating to surgeons and whether or not indemnity paid

absolute row % column % total %	indemnity yes	 no	 row total
surgeon			
	101	202	303
general	33,3	66,7	32,7
surgeon	29,1	34,9	
	10,9	21,8	
	54	95	149
orthopaedic	36,2	63,8	16,1
surgeon	15,6	16,4	
	5,8	10,3	
	24	34	58
oral surgeon	41,4	58,6	6,3
	6,9	5,9	
	2,6	3,7	
	8	10	18
cardio-	44,4	55,6	1,9
vascular	2,3	1,7	
surgeon	0,9	1,1	
		4	4
thoracic		100,0	0,4
surgeon		0,7	
		0,4	
	5	10	15
neuro	33,3	66,7	1,6
surgeon	1,4	1,7	
	0,5	1,1	
	11	22	33
plastic	33,3	66,7	3,6
surgeon	3,2	3,8	
	1,2	2,4	
surgeon			
	2	2	4
pediatric	50,0	50,0	0,4
surgeon	0,6	0,3	
	0,2	0,2	
	15	16	31
eye surgeon	48,4	51,6	3,3
	4,3	2,8	
	1,6	1,7	
	20	36	56
ENT doctor	35,7	64,3	6,0
	5,8	6,2	
	2,2	3,9	
	68	86	154
gynae-	44,2	55,8	16,6
cologist	19,6	14,9	
	7,3	9,3	
	18	32	50
urologist	36,0	64,0	5,4
	5,2	5,5	
	1,9	3,5	
	20	30	50
assistant	40,0	60,0	5,4
specialist	5,8	5,2	
	2,2	3,2	
	1		1
other	100,0		0,1
	0,3		
	0,1		
Column	347	579	926
Total	37,5	62,5	100,0

Valid cases: 926 Missing cases: 1

Table 39 Injury claims relating to non-surgical specialists and whether or not indemnity paid

absolute row % column % total %	indemnity yes	 no	row total
non-surgical specialist			
	18	32	50
specialist in	36,0	64,0	13,9
internal		13,0	14,4
disorders		5,0	8,9
		7	7
lung doctor		100,0	1,9
		3,2	
		1,9	
	1	16	17
cardiologist	5,9	94,1	4,7
	0,7	7,2	
	0,3	4,4	
		1	1
rheuma-		100,0	0,3
tologist		0,5	
		0,3	
	2	4	6
derma-	33,3	66,7	1,7
tologist	1,4	1,8	
	0,6	1,1	
	7	23	30
neurologist	23,3	76,7	8,3
	5,1	10,4	
	1,9	6,4	
		5	5
psychiatrist		100,0	1,4
		2,3	
		1,4	
	2	6	8
paediatrician	25,0	75,0	2,2
	1,4	2,7	
	0,6	1,7	

absolute row % column % total %	indemnity yes	 no	row total
non-surgical specialist			
	15	22	37
radiologist	40,5	59,5	10,3
	10,9	9,9	
	4,2	6,1	145
radio-	20,0	80,0	1,4
therapist	0,7	1,8	
	0,3	1,1	
	3	3	6
path.	50,0	50,0	1,7
anatomist	2,2	1,4	
	0,8	0,8	
	86	96	182
Anaesthetist	47,3	52,7	50,6
	62,3	43,2	
	23,9	26,7	
		1	1
rehabilitation		100,0	0,3
[centre]		0,5	
doctor		0,3	
		2	2
assistant		100,0	0,6
specialist		0,9	
		0,6	
	3		3
other	100,0		0,8
	2,2		
	0,8		
Column	138	222	360
Total	38,3	61,7	100,0

Valid cases: 360Missing cases: 0

Table 40 Injury claims relating to non-specialist doctors whether or not indemnity paid

absolute row % column % total %	**indemnity** yes	no	row total
	11	18	29
A+E doctor	37,9	62,1	69,0
	57,9	78,3	
	26,2	42,9	
	8	5	13
junior doctor	61,5	38,5	31,0
	42,1	21,7	
	19,0	11,9	
Column	19	23	42
Total	45,2	54,8	100,0

Valid cases: 42 Missing cases: 0

Table 41 Injury claims relating to other operators and whether or not indemnity paid

absolute row % column % total %	**Indemnity** yes	no	row total
other operators			
	1	5	6
obstetrician	16,7	83,3	3,8
	1,0	8,2	
	0,6	3,2	
	3	1	4
radiographer	75,0	25,0	2,5
	3,1	1,6	
	1,9	0,6	
	1	4	5
physio-	20,0	80,0	3,2
therapist	1,0	6,6	
	0,6	2,5	
	41	38	79
nurse	51,9	48,1	50,0
	42,3	62,3	
	25,9	24,1	
other operators			
	1		1
house	100,0		0,6
officcr	1,0		
	0,6		
	46	12	58
analyst	79,3	20,7	36,7
	47,4	19,7	
	29,1	7,6	
	4	1	5
other	80,0	20,0	3,2
	4,1	1,6	
	2,5	0,6	
Column	97	61	158
Total	61,4	38,6	100,0

Valid cases: 158 Missing cases: 0

Table 42 Injury claims by year reported and by operators

absolute row % column % total %	surgeon	non-surgical operator	non-specialist doctors	other	no operator	row total
Year reported						
1980	5	2	1	1		9
	55,6	22,2	11,1	11,1		0,6
	0,5	0,6	2,4	0,6		
	0,3	0,1	0,1	0,1		
1981	15	3		2		20
	75,0	15,0	10,0		1,3	
	1,6	0,8	1,3			
	1,0	0,2	0,1			
1982	28	10	1	6		45
	62,2	22,2	2,2	13,3		3,0
	3,0	2,8	2,4	3,8		
	1,9	0,7	0,1	0,4		
1983	53	29	1	12	2	97
	54,6	29,9	1,0	12,4	2,1	6,5
	5,7	8.1	2,4	7,6	18,2	
	3,5	1,9	0,1	0.8	0,1	
1984	86	41	6	12	2	147
	58,5	27,9	4.1	8,2	1,4	9,8
	9,3	11,4	14,3	7,6	18,2	
	5,7	2,7	0,4	0,8	0,1	
1985	104	43	3	14	3	167
	62,3	25.7	1,8	8,4	1,8	11,1
	11,2	11,9	7,1	8,9	27,3	
	6,9	2,9	0,2	0,9	0.2	
1986	134	41	6	15	2	198
	67,7	20,7	3,0	7,6	1,0	13,2
	14,5	11,4	14,3	9,5	18,2	
	8,9	2,7	0,4	1,0	0,1	
1987	122	41	6	16		185
	65,9	22,2	3,2	8,6		12,3
	13,2	11,4	14,3	10,1		
	8,1	2,7	0,4	1,1		
1988	171	49	10	71	1	302
	56.6	16,2	3,3	23,5	0,3	20.2
	18,4	13,6	23,8	44,9	9,1	
	11,4	3,3	0,7	4,7	0,1	
1989	209	101	8	9	1	328
	63,7	30,8	2,4	2,7	0,3	21,9
	22,5	28,1	19,0	5,7	9,1	
	14,0	6,7	0,5	0.6	0,1	
Column	927	360	42	158	11	1498
Total	61,9	24,0	2,8	10,5	0,7	100,0

Valid cases: 1498 Missing cases: 52

Table 43 Injury claims by medico-technical basis

	number	%	valid %
incorrect/late diagnosis	192	12,4	12,5
other diagnosis-related aspects	15	1,0	1,0
incorrect medication	22	1,4	1,4
incorrect blood/other fluids	12	0,8	0,8
other medication-related aspects	5	1,0	1,0
incorrect anaesthetic	7	0,5	0,5
intubation technique	111	7,2	7,3
other anaesthetic-related aspects	7	1,1	1,1
incorrect technico-surgical procedure	343	22,1	22,4
positioning of body during operation	38	2,5	2,5
procedure not indicated	69	4,5	4,5
operating material accidentally left *in situ*	45	2,9	2,9
unsuccessful sterilisation	21	1,4	1,4
other operation-related aspects	87	5,6	5,7
incorrect/late delivery	17	1,1	1,1
other confinement-related aspects	19	1,2	1,2
injection/infusion/puncture techniques	120	7,7	7,8
catheterisation/internal exam.	45	2,9	2,9
incorrect dressings/splints etc.	63	4,1	4,1
infection	71	4,6	4,6
other medical reasons	40	2,6	2,6
no medical basis	162	10,5	10,6
not known	19	12	missing
Total	1550	100,0	100,0

Valid cases: 1531 Missing cases: 19

Table 44 Injury claims by medico-technical basis and whether or not indemnity paid

absolute row % column %	**indemnity** yes	no	row total
medico-technical reason			
incorrect/late diagnosis	69	123	192
	35,9	64,1	12,5
	11,1	13,6	
other diagnosis-related aspects	8	7	15
	53,3	46,7	1,0
	1,3	0,8	
incorrect medication	12	10	22
	54,5	45,5	1,4
	1,9	1,1	
incorrect blood/other fluids	7	5	12
	58,3	41,7	0,8
		1,1	0,6
other medication-related aspects	3	12	15
	20,0	80,0	1,0
	0.5	1,3	
incorrect anaesthetic	3	4	7
	42,9	57,1	0,5
	0,5	0,4	
intubation technique	67	44	111
	60,4	39,6	7,3
	10,7	4,9	
other anaesthetic-related aspects	6	11	17
	35,5	64,7	1,1
	1,0	1,2	
incorrect technico-surgical procedure	122	220	342
	35,7	64,3	22,4
	19,6	24,3	
positioning of body during operation/ anaesthetic	15	23	38
	39,5	60,5	2,5
	2,4	2,5	
procedure not indicated	34	35	69
	49,3	50,7	4,5
	5,4	3,9	

continued on page 79 ▸

absolute row % column %	indemnity yes	no	row total
medico-technical reason			
operating material	33	12	45
accidentally left	73,3	26,7	2,9
in situ	5,3	1,3	
unsuccessful sterilisation	9	12	21
	42,9	57,1	1,4
	1,4	1,3	
other operation-related	17	70	87
aspects	19,5	80,5	5,7
	2,7	7,7	
incorrect/late delivery	8	9	17
	47,1	52,9	1,1
	1,3	1,0	
other confinement-related	8	11	19
aspects	42,1	57,9	1,2
	1,3	1,2	
injection/infusion/	43	77	120
puncture techniques	35,8	64,2	7,8
	6,9	8,5	
catheterisation/internal	11	34	45
exam.	24,4	75,6	2,9
	1,8	3,8	
incorrect dressings/	24	39	63
splints	38,1	61,9	4,1
	3,8	4,3	
infection	51	20	71
	71,8	28,2	4,6
	8,2	2,2	
other medical reasons	18	22	40
	45,0	55,0	2,6
	2,9	2,4	
no medical basis	56	106	162
	34,6	65,4	10,6
	9,0	11,7	
Column	624	906	1530
Total	40,8	59,2	100,0

Valid cases: 1530 Missing observations: 20

Table 45 Injury claims by basis of general aspects of treatment

	number	%	valid %
Doctor's delay	15	1,0	4,7
incorrect treatment protocol	69	4,5	21,6
inadequate result of treatment	45	2,9	14,1
incorrect follow-up/supervision	59	3,8	18,5
discourtesy	27	1,7	8,5
incorrect nursing/care	62	4,0	19,4
other	42	2,7	13,2
not known/n/a	1231	79,4	missing
Total	1550	100,0	100,0

Valid cases: 319 Missing cases: 1231

Table 46 Injury claims by basis of general aspects of treatment and whether or not indemnity paid

absolute row % column %	indemnity yes	 no	 row total
general aspects			
doctor's delay	4	11	15
	26,7	73,3	4,7
	4,8	4,7	
incorrect treatment protocol	28	41	69
	40,6	59,4	21,6
	33,3	17,4	
inadequate result of treatment	5	40	45
	11,1	88,9	14,1
	6,0	17,0	
incorrect follow-up or supervision	14	45	59
	23,7	76,3	18,5
	16,7	19,1	
discourtesy	4	23	27
	14,8	85,2	8,5
	4,8	9,8	
incorrect nursing/care	19	43	62
	30,6	69,4	19,4
	22,6	18,3	
other	10	32	42
	23,8	76,2	13,2
	11,9	13,6	
Column	84	235	319
Total	26,3	73,7	100,0

Valid cases: 319 Missing cases: 1231

Table 47 Injury claims by basis of medical equipment

	number	%	valid %
incorrect use	46	3,0	25,1
defective equipment	22	1,4	12,0
incorrect use and/or defective equipment	111	7,2	60,7
other aspects	4	0,3	2,2
not known/n/a	1367	88,2	missing
Total	1550	100,0	100,0

Valid cases: 183 Missing cases: 1367

Table 48 Injury claims by basis of medical equipment used and whether or not indemnity paid

absolute row % column % total %	indemnity yes	 no	 row total
basis: medical equipment			
incorrect use	27 58,7 22,1 14,8	19 41,3 31,1 10,4	46 25,1
defective equipment	13 59,1 10,7 7,1	9 40,9 14,8 4,9	22 12,0
incorrect use and/ or defective equipment	79 71,2 64,8 43,2	32 28,8 52,5 17,5	111 60,7
other aspects	3 75,0 2,5 1,6	1 25,0 1,6 0,5	4 2,2
Column Total	122 66,7	61 33,3	183 100,0

Valid cases: 183 Missing cases: 1367

Table 49 Injury claims by basis of lack of consent or insufficient information

	number	%	valid %
no/insufficient consent	22	1,4	22,9
incorrect/insufficient information	69	4,5	71,9
other	5	0,3	5,2
not known/n/a	1454	93,8	missing
Total	1550	100,0	100,0

Valid cases: 96 Missing cases: 1454

Table 50 Injury claims by lack of consent or insufficient information and whether or not indemnity paid

absolute row % column %	**indemnity** yes	no	row total
formal aspects			
no/insufficient consent	5	17	22
	22,7	77,3	22,9
	19,2	24,3	
incorrect/insufficient	20	49	69
information	29,0	71,0	71,9
	76,9	70,0	
other	1	4	5
	20,0	80,0	5,2
	3,8	5,7	
Column	26	70	96
Total	27,1	72,9	100,0

Valid cases: 96 Missing cases: 1454

Table 51 Injury claims by type of injury

	number	%	valid %
dental lesion	148	9,5	9,9
burns etc.	133	8,6	8,9
(partial) amputation	35	2,3	2,3
facial nerve lesions	22	1,4	1,5
other external injury	6	0,4	0,4
functional/nervous disorders of limbs	383	24,7	25,6
transverse lesion	15	1,0	1,0
fracture	27	1,7	1,8
functional disorder of lung	23	1,5	1,5
functional disorder of urinary tract	35	2,3	2,3
functional disorder of kidney	7	0,5	0,5
functional disorder of stomach/intestine/oesophagus	44	2,8	2,9
functional disorder of sexual organ	19	1,2	1,3
functional disorder of vocal chord	11	0,7	0,7
functional disorder of other organs	24	1,5	1,6
(partial) removal of organs	18	1,2	1,2
functional disorder of ear	13	0,8	0,9
functional disorder of eye	40	2,6	2,7
functional disorder of other sense-organs	4	0,3	0,3
death	54	3,5	3,6
pregnancy	22	1,4	1,5
cerebral infarct	10	0,6	0,7
coma	1	0,1	0,1
brain damage	7	0,5	0,5
inflammation/infection	103	6,6	6,9
pain/discomfort	228	14,7	15,2
psychic trauma	22	1,4	1,5
financial loss	11	0,7	0,7
other injuries	24	1,5	1,6
not known	61	4,0	missing
Total	1550	100,0	100,0

Valid cases: 1489 Missing cases: 61

Table 52 Injury claims by type of injury and whether or not indemnity paid

absolute row % column %	indemnity yes	 no	 row total
injury			
dental lesion	89	59	148
	60,1	39,9	9,9
	14,3	6,8	
burns etc.	82	51	133
	61,7	38,3	8,9
	13,1	5,8	
(partial) amputation	15	20	35
	42,9	57,1	2,3
	2,4	2,3	
facial nerve lesions	5	16	21
	23,8	76,2	1,4
	0,8	1,8	
other external injury	1	5	6
	16,7	83,3	0,4
	0,2	0,6	
functional/nervous disorder of limbs	140	243	383
	36,6	63,4	25,6
	22,4	27,8	
transverse lesion	5	10	15
	33,3	66,7	1,0
	0,8	1,1	
fracture	14	13	27
	51,9	48,1	1,8
	2,2	1,5	
functional disorder of lung	7	16	23
	30,4	69,6	1,5
	1,1	1,8	
functional disorder of urinary tract	16	19	36
	45,7	54,3	2,3
	2,6	2,2	
functional disorder of kidney	3	4	7
	42,9	57,1	0,5
	0,5	0,5	

continued on page 85 ▸

absolute row % column %	**indemnity** yes	no	row total
injury			
functional disorder of stomach/intestine/oesophagus	23 52,3 3,7	21 47,7 2,4	44 2,9
functional disorder of sexual organ	4 21,1 0,6	15 78,9 1,7	19 1,3
functional disorder of vocal chords	1 9,1 0,2	10 90,9 1,1	11 0,7
functional disorder of other organs	8 33,3 1,3	16 66,7 1,8	24 1,6
(partial) removal of organs	5 27,8 0,8	13 72,2 1,5	18 1,2
functional disorder of ear	3 23,1 0,5	10 76,9 1,1	13 0,9
functional disorder of eye	13 32,5 2,1	27 67,5 3,1	40 2,7
functional disorder of other sense-organs	3 75,0 0,5	1 25,0 0,1	4 0,3
death	9 16,7 1,4	45 83,3 5,2	54 3,6
pregnancy	7 31,8 1,1	15 68,2 1,7	22 1,5
cerebral infarct	3 30,0 0,5	7 70,0 0,8	10 0,7

continued on page 86 ▸

absolute row % column %	indemnity yes	 no	 row total
injury			
coma		1	1
		100,0	0,1
		0,1	
brain damage	6	1	7
	85,7	14,3	0,5
	1,0	0,1	
inflammation/infection	53	50	103
	51,5	48,5	6,9
	8,5	5,7	
pain/discomfort	84	144	228
	36,8	63,2	15,2
	13,5	16,5	
psychic trauma	7	15	22
	31,8	68,2	1,5
	1,1	1,7	
financial loss	8	3	11
	72,7	27,3	0,7
	1,3	0,3	
other injuries	8	16	24
	33,3	66,7	1,6
	1,3	1,8	
Column Total	622 41,7	866 58,3	1488 100,0

Valid cases: 1488 Missing cases: 62

Appendix 2

DESCRIPTION OF INDEMNITIES OF *f* 100,000.-- AND ABOVE

1. Total loss of function of left inner ear after ENT operation on facial nerve. The female patient (aged 32 years) has the following symptoms: total failure of left organ of equilibrium, total deafness in left ear, and also giddiness.

   As a result of this, the patient is entirely incapable of working (she was formerly a waitress in a cafeteria).

   Liability has been admitted.

   Two neutral expert physicians' reports contradict one another as regards the improvement to be anticipated in balance (by compensation on the part of the right organ of equilibrium) and in respect of the consequences this will have on the patient's capacity or incapacity to work.

   The third neutral expert physician consulted believes that the patient is totally incapable of work and can perform only light household tasks. Furthermore, cycling and driving are possible to a very limited extent only. Some improvement in balance may still occur. Incapacity is estimated at 18% (AMA) of the whole person.

   In consultation with the patient's legal advisor total damages have been set ad *f* 115,000.--, *f* 17,500.-- of which is in respect of compensation for pain and suffering.

2. Female patient (aged 50) admitted for a neurosurgical operation.

   Subcutaneous oedema developed after an infusion was incorrectly applied (anaesthetic). A second operation appeared to be necessary. Examination has shown that the arm of the patient (a saleswoman) is now totally non-functional. Incapacity is estimated at 60% (AMA) of the whole person.
   Liability has been admitted.
   Compensation totalling approximately *f* 105,000.-- has been agreed with the patient's legal advisor, *f* 30,000.-- of this being compensation for pain and suffering and *f* 45,000.-- for household assistance.

3. Following removal of a cyst in the jaw, a male patient (aged 52 years) ate a hard piece of bread which resulted in a fracture of the jaw. Occlusion of the lower and upper teeth is no longer good as a result of the fracture.

Liability has been admitted: the patient was not given instructions regarding eating. Compensation of 50% has been proposed, because some caution would also have been expected on the part of the patient.

In consultation with the patient's legal advisor (the patient is a musician), settlement was agreed for a sum of *f* 160,000.--, some *f* 25,000.-- of this being compensation for pain and suffering.

4. A male patient (26-year-old skilled construction worker) underwent surgery for ingrowing nails on both big toes. One of the two toes was subsequently bandaged too tightly resulting in slight necrosis. Plastic surgery is required. The toe is still very sensitive.

Liability has been admitted.

A neutral expert found additional stiffness and sensitivity of the toe in question. Incapacity is estimated at 3% of the whole person (AMA).

The Community Medical Service finds the patient totally incapable of work.

Compensation of approximately *f* 120,000.-- has been agreed with a legal aid insurer, approximately *f* 8,000.-- of this figure being compensation for pain and suffering.

The lost of income claim constitutes the most significant item of the indemnity.

5. A male patient (aged 47 years) was admitted because of nose-bleeds which could not be staunched. Sedative were prescribed because the patient was constantly restless. The patient subsequently became subcomatose and suffered cardiac arrest. After about 15 minutes in intensive care, the heart resumed functioning. As a result of this, the patient suffered brain damage. The wrong medicines had been prescribed. Moreover, there is also a claim of poor medical care in intensive care.

It was initially unclear which of the attending specialists acted negligently. Various mistakes were made. After the serving of writs by an advocate on both the hospitals and four specialists, the hospital insurer appears to be prepared to admit liability.

Examination by a neutral expert physician shows that the patient is totally incapable of work. The patient has his own business which has in the meantime failed. Damages have been set a *f* 640,000.-- in consultation with the patient's lawyer, *f* 75,000.-- of this being compensation for pain and suffering.

6. A male patient (aged 42 years) was given six courses of chemotherapy for the treatment of testicular cancer. After a number of chemotherapy courses, it was found that pulmonary metastasis was in remission. The specialist neglected to check whether metastasis had occurred elsewhere in the body. This incomplete diagnosis meant that it was only just possible to remove a substantial abdominal tumour in a late phase, which had caused considerable damage in the meantime.

   The patient lodged a complaint with the Medical Disciplinary Tribunal which served a warning order on the specialist involved.

   A neutral expert finds that the patient is totally incapable of work. As a result of various factors, the patient has disposed of his own business.

   Liability has been admitted. The question as to the extent to which the incapacity for work may be imputed to the incorrect treatment is the subject of a civil lawsuit. Furthermore, the patient has twice applied for an advance in short cause; one application was granted, the other rejected. As of the reference date (1.1.1991), the file is still open; in the meantime, the total advances paid out amount to approximately *f* 400,000.--.

7. A female patient (aged 48 years) had an indwelling epidural catheter inserted to combat pain. Clonic spasms developed as a result of incorrect administration and the incorrect use of various infused agents, resulting in fracture of both hips.

   Two hip protheses were subsequently inserted. A neutral expert physician has set incapacity at 50% of the whole person.

   Liability has been admitted.

   Compensation of approximately *f* 100,000.-- has been agreed with the patient's lawyer, *f* 50,000.-- of which is compensation for pain and suffering.

8. After an unsuccessful suicide attempt, a male patient (aged 38 years) was admitted to an internal medical ward where he was given a room to himself. After medication had been established, the patient appeared to be resting. His wife was afraid of another attempt at suicide but the attending specialist considered the situation to be less serious. Ultimately however, it was decided to admit the patient to the psychiatric ward. Just before he was due to be transferred, the patient jumped out of the window. As a result of this, he sustained serious injuries (various fractures, including a fractured hip).

Liability has been admitted. On the one hand, the attending specialist incorrectly assessed the patient's condition, on the other hand, the window of the room (3rd floor) could be opened too easily.

The patient is a self-employed businessman by profession and is claiming, in particular, for loss of income. Compensation of over *f* 600,000.-- has been agreed with patient's lawyer, *f* 100,000.-- of which is compensation for pain and suffering.

In the meantime the patient's sickness costs insurers have also submitted a claim. As of the reference date, a sum of approximately *f* 100,000.-- had been paid.

9. A female patient (aged 16 years) was admitted with serious injuries resulting from a road traffic accident. The patient was transferred directly to a larger hospital because there was a possible head injury, among other things. Not all the necessary diagnostic procedures were performed there. Moreover, the x-ray photograph was not assessed well. As a result, a dislocation high in the spine was not found and operated on promptly. This led to the development of a partial transverse lesion.

Discharge from hospital was followed by a long period of rehabilitation. Initial condylar necrosis of the right hip was not noticed at the rehabilitation centre, leading to the development of serious hip problems. Insofar as the hospital's insurer is the same as the insurer of the rehabilitation centre, the two files are considered as a single case for the purpose of the survey.

Liability has been admitted for both incidents.

The report from a neutral expert physician shows that the patient's total incapacity must be estimated at 70%. Without the transverse lesion, i.e. solely as a result of the accident, this would have been 10%.

The patient has been fully indemnified by the hospital insurers. The indemnity awarded amounted to *ƒ* 315,000.--, of which *ƒ* 75,000.-- was compensation for pain and suffering. The insurers have since brought a recourse action against the insurance company whose insured was (jointly) responsible for the motor accident. The latter company will ultimately contribute to the indemnity to the tune of 25%.

The sickness insurance fund is also making a claim. The hospital insurer will also pay 75% of this. Indemnification as of the reference date amounts to approximately *ƒ* 75,000.--.

10. A female patient (aged 54 years) was operated on for recurrent hernia. During the high-risk operation, a nerve root was irreparably damaged (with a chisel). As a result, the patient is largely wheelchair-bounded (serious functional impairment of the leg).

    Liability has ultimately been admitted.

    After laborious negotiations with the patient's lawyer, compensation in the sum of approximately *ƒ* 150,000.-- has been agreed, *ƒ* 60.000,-- of this being compensation for pain and suffering.

11. A twenty-six-year-old male primary school teacher was prescribed medication for the treatment of pleurisy and tuberculosis. As a result of taking these medicines, his sight was impaired. The patient was known to have eye problems. According to a neutral expert, the specialist made an error of judgement. He omitted to have an ophthalmological examination performed prior to prescribing the medication. Furthermore, the patient was not informed of the risks/side effects of the drugs.

    The patient began a civil action. The court rejected a claim for damages. The claim was granted on appeal.

    The expert report shows that is not possible to ascertain whether the medication contributed to the further deterioration of the eye condition. The court believes that this is a risk taken by the specialist. Incapacity, as a percentage, is unclear.

    After laborious negotiations, compensation in the sum of approximately *ƒ* 250,000.-- has been agreed, *ƒ* 65,000.-- of this being compensation for pain and suffering. The financial loss consists of reduced capacity to work and indemnification for household assistance.

12. A female patient (aged 33 years) underwent an abdominal operation which, on the basis of the reports, must be regarded as experimental. However, the patient appears in retrospect to have been absolutely unsuitable as a candidate. The operation had a series of serious sequelae, including total incontinence, partial aphasia and impaired ability to walk. More than a year later the patient died of these sequelae. Initially, the claim was rejected on the basis of the expert physician's report, which mentions complications for which no blame can be assigned. The patient's husband subsequently stated that there was no question of "informed consent".

Liability was then admitted.

Compensation of *f* 115,000.-- has been agreed with the claims settlement agency. In view of the fact that the claim for compensation in this case is based on Article 1406 Dutch Civil Code (death), no compensation for pain and suffering can be awarded.

13. A twenty-seven-year-old nurse became pregnant after having been sterilised. She gave birth to twins. During delivery by caesarian section, it was seen that the clips were not well attached to the Fallopian tubes.

Furthermore, the patient said that she had been inadequately advised of the risks of sterilisation.

Without liability being admitted, compensation of *f* 100,000.-- has been agreed with the patient's legal advisor and the claims settlement agency. The proportion accounted for by compensation for pain and suffering is unknown.

14. A hysterectomy was performed in the context of cancer of the womb, after which the female patient (aged 59 years) was given radiotherapy using a new method. This resulted in major damage being caused to the vagina and rectum, inter alia: a number of subsequent operations were necessary (including setting up a temporary stoma).

Liability has been admitted.

The patient used a civil action to claim higher compensation than had been offered. The court rejected the claim. Compensation of approximately *f* 130,000.-- has been agreed with the patient's lawyer, *f* 60,000.-- of this being compensation for pain and suffering.

15. The same case as above. As a result of incorrect radiotherapy, the

female patient has chronic pain, urinary incontinence and damage to the vagina and rectum. In this case, again, a number of subsequent operations followed (including setting up a temporary stoma).

Liability has been admitted.

Compensation of ƒ 110,000.-- has been agreed with a legal assistance insurer, ƒ 60,000.-- of this being compensation for pain and suffering.

16. A female patient (aged 63 years) was intubated in connection with a cataract operation. Pulmonary problems developed as a result of the intubation: septic shock and double pneumonia. The patient was kept in the ventilation centre for fourteen days. The patient has suffered serious functional impairment.

    Liability has been admitted for the fact that the anaesthetist intervened too late.

    Incapacity as a percentage is not known.

    Compensation of over ƒ 100,000.-- has been agreed with the patient's fourth legal advisor, ƒ 60,000.-- of this being compensation for pain and suffering.

17. A 19 year old notary's clerk underwent a knee operation in which a knee prosthesis was inserted. The patient was known to have had knee problems for many years previously, particularly with respect to stability. A period of rehabilitation followed the operation. The knee still appeared to be unstable. It was then mobilised (bending) under anaesthetic. This resulted in haemorrhage. Ultimately, the affected knee became dystrophic.

    Liability with respect to the mobilisation and the consequences thereof has been admitted. It is clear that major impairment would have occurred in this patient even without the incorrect procedure.

    The patient's legal assistance insurer claimed a high advance in short cause with respect to the loss of capacity to work. The claim was rejected. The causes of the dystrophy are still insufficiently clear.

    The court of appeal allowed the patient's claim. The advance was of ƒ 250,000.--.

    After laborious negotiations with both the lawyer and the claims settlement agency, damages have been set at approximately *f* 750,000.--. The amount of compensation for pain and suffering is unknown. The loss of capacity to work constitutes the largest item of the claim.

18. A thoracic vertebra was removed in a 47 year old company director. Post-operative signs of paralysis developed but were not noted. Surgical intervention therefore occurred too late. A transverse lesion had already developed as a result of haemorrhage in the spinal cord.

    Liability has been admitted.

    The patient's legal advisor has begun a civil action to establish the extent of compensation. The claim is for *f* 800,000.--, *f* 130,000.-- of this being compensation for pain and suffering. As of the reference date a sum of *f* 100,000.-- has been paid out in advances.

19. A male patient (aged 52 years) was operated on for a cervical cyst. During the operation, it appeared that they were dealing with a vascular tumour instead of a cyst. Post-operative haemorrhage occurred resulting in hemiparesis.

    Liability has been admitted. On finding the vascular tumour, the general surgeon should have passed the operation on to a different specialist.

    Compensation of almost *f* 110,000.-- has been agreed with the lawyer, *f* 75,000.-- of this being compensation for pain and suffering.

20. A female patient (aged 25 years) was admitted with threatened labour (seven months). Medication was administered to stop the contractions. The patient was also isolated. A long period of vomiting followed (post-cerebral-oedema status as a result of (pre-)eclampsia). A caesarian section was performed after ten days. The patient lost consciousness and was ventilated for seven weeks. As a result of this, the patient suffered brain damage. A neutral expert estimates the permanent incapacity at 80%.

    Liability has been admitted as regards inadequate supplementing with vitamin B, a shortage of which developed as a result of the long period of vomiting.
    The patient's husband has lodged a complaint with the Medical Disciplinary Tribunal. Insofar as the complaint applies to the gynaecologist, it has been upheld. With regard to the anaesthetist, the complaint was dismissed.

Compensation in the sum of ƒ 225,000.-- has been agreed with the lawyer, ƒ 75,000.-- of which is compensation for pain and suffering.

Overall description of cases of above ƒ 100,000.--

Those claims for compensation in which ƒ 100,000.-- or above was paid out were considered in more detail from a number of aspects for the purpose of comparison. The most remarkable differences from the picture which emerged from the survey of all the claims (n = 1550) are described below. The value is given, incidentally, with reference to the largest claims (n = 20), followed by the value obtained in the survey of all the injury claims (n = 1550).

In all the twenty cases it is apparent that there has been legal assistance (100% as against 60%). This fact underlines the supposition that the greater the loss and/or the injury as a result of an incorrect procedure in hospital, the more likely the patient is to enlist legal assistance. Moreover, in five cases a civil action appears to have been instituted (25% as against 4%) while in two cases a complaint was lodged with a medical disciplinary tribunal (20% as against 6%).

Furthermore, we see that in fifteen cases of claims with indemnities of ƒ 100,000.-- or above, a neutral expert physician was consulted (75% as against 20%). In six cases, the opinion given was with regard to establishing the percentage of permanent incapacity (40% as against 17%), while in eight of the other nine cases an opinion was given with reference to whether or not actions were in accordance with good medical practice and/or to a causal connection (53% as against 67%). In one case, the neutral expert gave an opinion, on the one hand, as to whether or not actions were in accordance with good medical practice and/or whether a causal connection existed, and, on the other, he established the percentage of permanent incapacity (7% as against 14%). We can see that, proportionally, more neutral experts were consulted to assess the degree of permanent incapacity. It is likely that this is connected with the complexity of the degree and extent of the injury. Permanent injury appears to be involved in fifteen cases among the largest claims for compensation (75%).
As regards the operators involved in the incorrect procedures, it would appear that in these cases the category of "surgeons" (45% as against 62%) is the same size as that of non-surgical specialists (45% as against 24%). Two of the remaining cases involve several specialists and in one case the operator involved was a nurse.